Pediatric Airway Management

for the Prehospital Professional

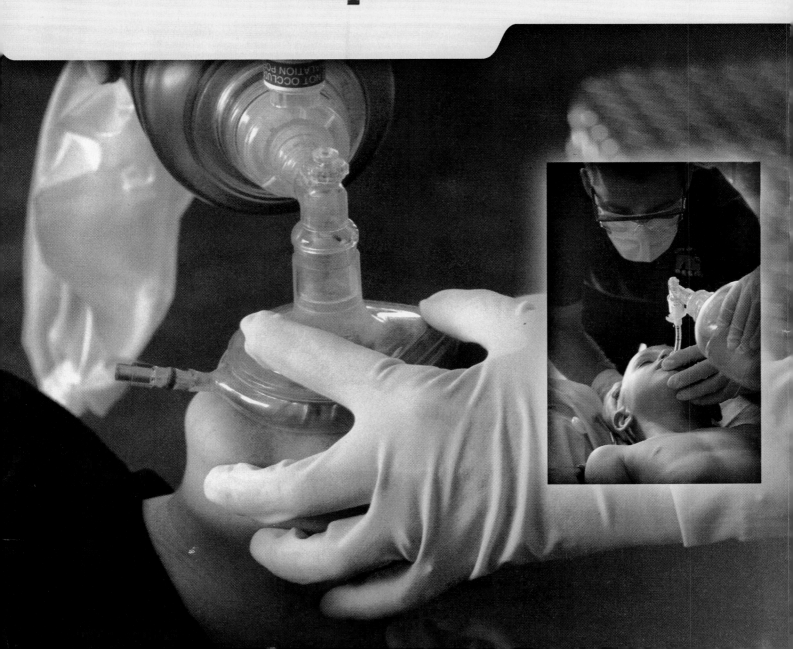

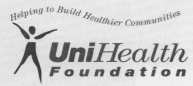

Supported by a grant from UniHealth Foundation, a non-profit philanthropic organization whose mission is to support and facilitate activities that significantly improve the health and well being of individuals and communities within its service area.

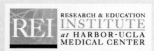

Research & Education Institute at Harbor-UCLA Medical Center

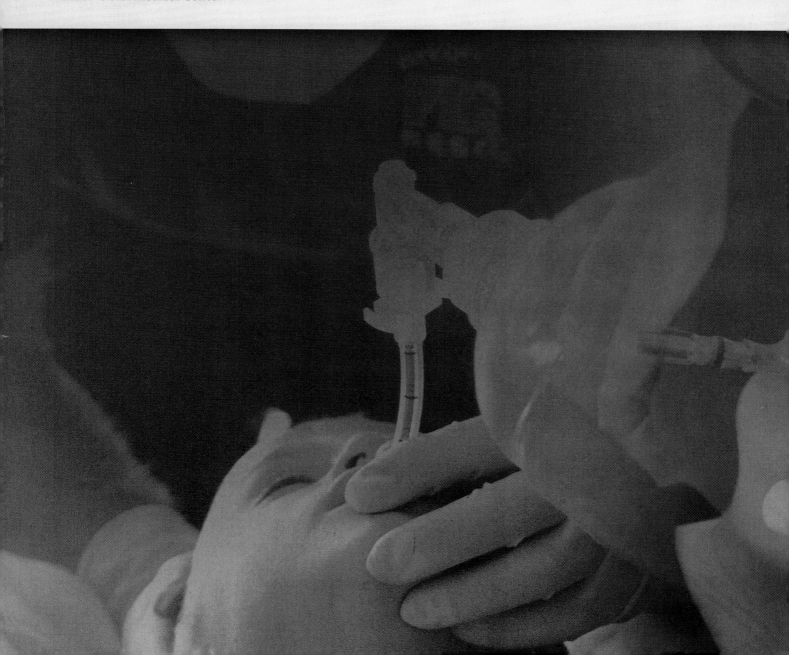

Pediatric
Airway
Management
for the Prehospital Professional

Marianne Gausche-Hill, MD, FACEP, FAAP
Professor of Medicine
David Geffen School of Medicine at UCLA
Director, EMS and EMS Fellowship
Director, Pediatric Emergency Medicine Fellowship
Harbor-UCLA Medical Center, Department of Emergency Medicine
Director, Pediatric Emergency Medicine, Little Company of Mary Hospital

Deborah P. Henderson, RN, PhD
Adjunct Associate Professor
Department of Pediatrics
David Geffen School of Medicine at UCLA
Co-Director, EMSC, Resource Alliance, Harbor-UCLA Medical Center

Suzanne M. Goodrich, RN, MSN
EMS Manager
City of Orange Fire Department

William Koenig, MD, FACEP
EMS Medical Director
Los Angeles County Department of Health Services
Medical Director, Mercy Air Service

Pamela Doil-Poore, RN
Emergency Department, Kona Community Hospital

JONES AND BARTLETT PUBLISHERS
Sudbury, Massachusetts
BOSTON   TORONTO   LONDON   SINGAPORE

World Headquarters
40 Tall Pine Drive
Sudbury, MA 01776
978-443-5000
info@jbpub.com
www.jbpub.com

Jones and Bartlett Publishers
Canada
2406 Nikanna Rd.
Mississauga, ON
Canada L5C 2W6

Jones and Bartlett Publishers
International
Barb House, Barb Mews
London W6 7PA
UK

Production Credits
Chief Executive Officer: Clayton E. Jones
Chief Operating Officer: Donald W. Jones, Jr.
President: Robert W. Holland, Jr.
V.P., Sales and Marketing: William Kane
V.P., Design and Production: Anne Spencer
V.P., Manufacturing and Inventory Control: Therese Bräuer
Publisher, Public Safety: Kimberly Brophy
Associate Managing Editor: Carol E. Brewer
Associate Managing Editor: Jennifer Reed
Production Editor: Scarlett L. Stoppa
Director, Marketing: Alisha Weisman
Director, Interactive Technology: Adam Alboyadjian
Interactive Technology Manager: Dawn Mahon Priest
Text Design: Anne Spencer
Cover Design: Kristin Ohlin
Composition: Graphic World
Printing and Binding: Courier Kendallville
Cover Printer: Phoenix Color

The procedures and protocols in this book are based on the most current recommendations of responsible medical sources. The publisher, however, makes no guarantee as to, and assumes no responsibility for the correctness, sufficiency or completeness of such information or recommendations. Other or additional safety measures may be required under particular circumstances.

This textbook is intended solely as a guide to the appropriate procedures to be employed when rendering emergency care to the sick and injured. It is not intended as a statement of the standards of care required in any particular situation, because circumstances and the patient's physical condition can vary widely from one emergency to another. Nor is it intended that this textbook shall in any way advise emergency personnel concerning legal authority to perform the activities or procedures discussed. Such local determinations should be made only with the aid of legal counsel.

Library of Congress Cataloging-in-Publication Data
Pediatric airway management / Marianne Gausche-Hill ... [et al.].-- 1st ed.
     p. ; cm.
  Includes index.
  ISBN 0-7637-2066-6 (pbk. : alk. paper)
  1. Respiratory therapy for children. 2. Airway (Medicine) 3. Lungs--Diseases, Obstructive. 4. Trachea--Intubation.
  [DNLM: 1. Airway Obstruction--Child. 2. Airway Obstruction--Infant. 3. Intubation--methods. WF 140 P3713 2004] I. Gausche-Hill, Marianne.
  RJ434.P43 2004
  618.92'2--dc22

                              2004003173

Additional credits appear on page 146, which constitutes a continuation of the copyright page.
Printed in the United States of America
08 07 06 05 04   10 9 8 7 6 5 4 3 2 1

Contents

Contents

Chapter 9: Special Needs: Tracheostomy 117

Contents

Pediatric Airway Management for the Prehospital Professional
is a complete, integrated learning system comprised of this text,
an Instructor's ToolKit CD-ROM, a DVD video, and an online
course. This one-of-a-kind learning system gives EMS providers
an opportunity to learn and practice critical pediatric airway
management skills.

Textbook Features

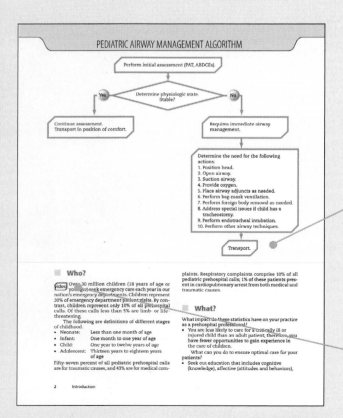

Scenario—Each chapter opens with a scenario to get the student thinking about how to handle this type of pediatric airway emergency.

CHAPTER 1

Introduction

Scenario

You are called to the home of a 4-year-old girl with a history of "choking." The mother called 9-1-1 and was given instructions by a dispatcher about how to deliver first aid to her unconscious child; she performed abdominal thrusts without relief of the obstruction.

When you arrive on scene, the patient is unconscious, there is no chest rise, and her skin is cyanotic.

1. What are your management priorities?
2. What anatomical, physiological, and behavioral factors may have led to this child's condition?

Think about these questions and this case as you read on. We will return to this scenario at the end of the chapter.

PEDIATRIC AIRWAY MANAGEMENT ALGORITHM

Perform initial assessment (PAT, ABDCEs).

Determine physiologic state. Stable?

Yes → Continue assessment. Transport in position of comfort.

No → Requires immediate airway management.

Determine the need for the following actions:
1. Position head.
2. Open airway.
3. Suction airway.
4. Provide oxygen.
5. Place airway adjuncts as needed.
6. Perform bag-mask ventilation.
7. Perform foreign body removal as needed.
8. Address special issues if child has a tracheostomy.
9. Perform endotracheal intubation.
10. Perform other airway techniques.

Transport.

Pediatric Airway Management Algorithm—Teaches the process for assessing and managing any pediatric airway emergency. Each chapter describes a different component of this invaluable tool.

■ Who?

Over 30 million children (18 years of age or younger) seek emergency care each year in our nation's emergency departments. Children represent 30% of emergency department patient visits. By contrast, children represent only 10% of all prehospital calls. Of these calls less than 5% are limb- or life-threatening.

The following are definitions of different stages of childhood.
- Neonate: Less than one month of age
- Infant: One month to one year of age
- Child: One year to twelve years of age
- Adolescent: Thirteen years to eighteen years of age

Fifty-seven percent of all pediatric prehospital calls are for traumatic causes, and 43% are for medical com-

plaints. Respiratory complaints comprise 10% of all pediatric prehospital calls; 1% of these patients present in cardiopulmonary arrest from both medical and traumatic causes.

■ What?

What impact do these statistics have on your practice as a prehospital professional?
- You are less likely to care for a critically ill or injured child than an adult patient; therefore, you have fewer opportunities to gain experience in the care of children.

What can you do to ensure optimal care for your patients?
- Seek out education that includes cognitive (knowledge), affective (attitudes and behaviors),

2   Introduction

Video link icon—Marks content that is also covered in the Pediatric Airway Management DVD.

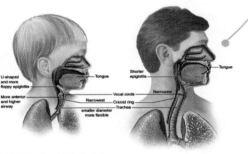

Figure 1-1 A child's airway is anatomically different than that of an adult.

Where's the Evidence?—These boxes provide a quick synopsis of the literature and efficacy of the techniques and management trends discussed in the chapter.

Full Color Anatomic Illustrations—This high-quality art makes it easy to understand the how's and why's.

Figure References—Appear in orange so they are easily seen.

Full Color Photos—Many depict real-life pediatric airway emergencies in the field and hospital settings.

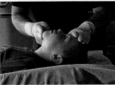

Figure 3-1 Head tilt-chin lift maneuver to open the airway.

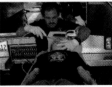

Figure 3-3 Suction the airway.

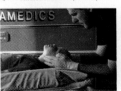

Figure 3-2 Jaw-thrust maneuver to open the airway.

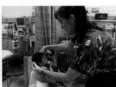

Figure 3-4 Provide supplemental oxygen.

Features

Tricks of the Trade—These boxes provide brief airway management tips gained from experience in the field.

Vocabulary Terms—Vocabulary terms appear in red and are underlined, alerting the reader that the term is defined at the end of the chapter and in the glossary.

Skill Drills—Step-by-step explanations and photos show how to perform pediatric airway management skills.

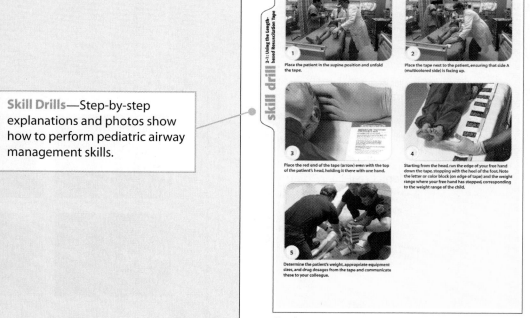

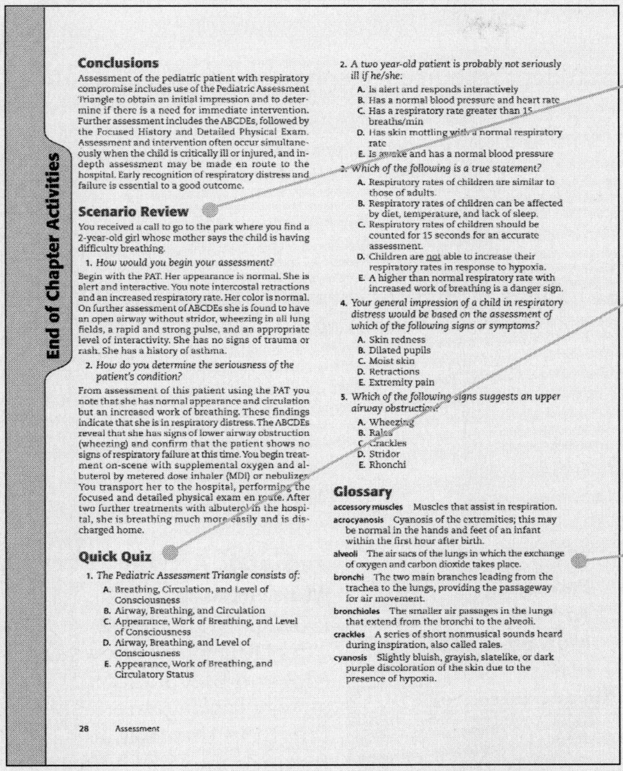

Page image content (sample chapter page)

Conclusions

Assessment of the pediatric patient with respiratory compromise includes use of the Pediatric Assessment Triangle to obtain an initial impression and to determine if there is a need for immediate intervention. Further assessment includes the ABCDEs, followed by the Focused History and Detailed Physical Exam. Assessment and intervention often occur simultaneously when the child is critically ill or injured, and in-depth assessment may be made en route to the hospital. Early recognition of respiratory distress and failure is essential to a good outcome.

Scenario Review

You received a call to go to the park where you find a 2-year-old girl whose mother says the child is having difficulty breathing.

1. How would you begin your assessment?

Begin with the PAT. Her appearance is normal. She is alert and interactive. You note intercostal retractions and an increased respiratory rate. Her color is normal. On further assessment of ABCDEs she is found to have an open airway without stridor, wheezing in all lung fields, a rapid and strong pulse, and an appropriate level of interactivity. She has no signs of trauma or rash. She has a history of asthma.

2. How do you determine the seriousness of the patient's condition?

From assessment of this patient using the PAT you note that she has normal appearance and circulation but an increased work of breathing. These findings indicate that she is in respiratory distress. The ABCDEs reveal that she has signs of lower airway obstruction (wheezing) and confirm that the patient shows no signs of respiratory failure at this time. You begin treatment on-scene with supplemental oxygen and albuterol by metered dose inhaler (MDI) or nebulizer. You transport her to the hospital, performing the focused and detailed physical exam en route. After two further treatments with albuterol in the hospital, she is breathing much more easily and is discharged home.

Quick Quiz

1. The Pediatric Assessment Triangle consists of:
  A. Breathing, Circulation, and Level of Consciousness
  B. Airway, Breathing, and Circulation
  C. Appearance, Work of Breathing, and Level of Consciousness
  D. Airway, Breathing, and Level of Consciousness
  E. Appearance, Work of Breathing, and Circulatory Status

2. A two year-old patient is probably not seriously ill if he/she:
  A. Is alert and responds interactively
  B. Has a normal blood pressure and heart rate
  C. Has a respiratory rate greater than 15 breaths/min
  D. Has skin mottling with a normal respiratory rate
  E. Is awake and has a normal blood pressure

3. Which of the following is a true statement?
  A. Respiratory rates of children are similar to those of adults.
  B. Respiratory rates of children can be affected by diet, temperature, and lack of sleep.
  C. Respiratory rates of children should be counted for 15 seconds for an accurate assessment.
  D. Children are not able to increase their respiratory rates in response to hypoxia.
  E. A higher than normal respiratory rate with increased work of breathing is a danger sign.

4. Your general impression of a child in respiratory distress would be based on the assessment of which of the following signs or symptoms?
  A. Skin redness
  B. Dilated pupils
  C. Moist skin
  D. Retractions
  E. Extremity pain

5. Which of the following signs suggests an upper airway obstruction?
  A. Wheezing
  B. Rales
  C. Crackles
  D. Stridor
  E. Rhonchi

Glossary

accessory muscles Muscles that assist in respiration.

acrocyanosis Cyanosis of the extremities; this may be normal in the hands and feet of an infant within the first hour after birth.

alveoli The air sacs of the lungs in which the exchange of oxygen and carbon dioxide takes place.

bronchi The two main branches leading from the trachea to the lungs, providing the passageway for air movement.

bronchioles The smaller air passages in the lungs that extend from the bronchi to the alveoli.

crackles A series of short nonmusical sounds heard during inspiration, also called rales.

cyanosis Slightly bluish, grayish, slatelike, or dark purple discoloration of the skin due to the presence of hypoxia.

28   Assessment

Scenario Review—A summary and answers to the scenario presented at the beginning of the chapter.

Quick Quiz—Test your knowledge with this brief multiple-choice quiz presented at the end of each chapter. Answers are found in the back of the text.

Vocabulary—Each chapter contains a list of vocabulary terms. A glossary is also provided at the end of the text.

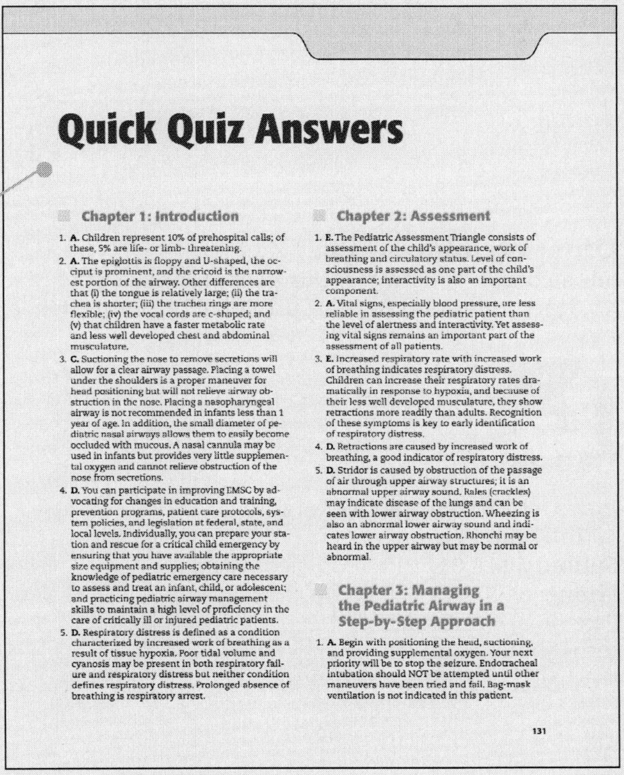

Quick Quiz Answers—This appendix provides the answers to the Quick Quizzes at the end of each chapter.

Quick Quiz Answers

Chapter 1: Introduction

1. **A.** Children represent 10% of prehospital calls; of these, 5% are life- or limb-threatening.

2. **A.** The epiglottis is floppy and U-shaped, the occiput is prominent, and the cricoid is the narrowest portion of the airway. Other differences are that (i) the tongue is relatively large; (ii) the trachea is shorter; (iii) the tracheal rings are more flexible; (iv) the vocal cords are c-shaped; and (v) that children have a faster metabolic rate and less well developed chest and abdominal musculature.

3. **C.** Suctioning the nose to remove secretions will allow for a clear airway passage. Placing a towel under the shoulders is a proper maneuver for head positioning but will not relieve airway obstruction in the nose. Placing a nasopharyngeal airway is not recommended in infants less than 1 year of age. In addition, the small diameter of pediatric nasal airways allows them to easily become occluded with mucous. A nasal cannula may be used in infants but provides very little supplemental oxygen and cannot relieve obstruction of the nose from secretions.

4. **D.** You can participate in improving EMSC by advocating for changes in education and training, prevention programs, patient care protocols, system policies, and legislation at federal, state, and local levels. Individually, you can prepare your station and rescue for a critical child emergency by ensuring that you have available the appropriate size equipment and supplies; obtaining the knowledge of pediatric emergency care necessary to assess and treat an infant, child, or adolescent; and practicing pediatric airway management skills to maintain a high level of proficiency in the care of critically ill or injured pediatric patients.

5. **D.** Respiratory distress is defined as a condition characterized by increased work of breathing as a result of tissue hypoxia. Poor tidal volume and cyanosis may be present in both respiratory failure and respiratory distress but neither condition defines respiratory distress. Prolonged absence of breathing is respiratory arrest.

Chapter 2: Assessment

1. **E.** The Pediatric Assessment Triangle consists of assessment of the child's appearance, work of breathing and circulatory status. Level of consciousness is assessed as one part of the child's appearance; interactivity is also an important component.

2. **A.** Vital signs, especially blood pressure, are less reliable in assessing the pediatric patient than the level of alertness and interactivity. Yet assessing vital signs remains an important part of the assessment of all patients.

3. **E.** Increased respiratory rate with increased work of breathing indicates respiratory distress. Children can increase their respiratory rates dramatically in response to hypoxia, and because of their less well developed musculature, they show retractions more readily than adults. Recognition of these symptoms is key to early identification of respiratory distress.

4. **D.** Retractions are caused by increased work of breathing, a good indicator of respiratory distress.

5. **D.** Stridor is caused by obstruction of the passage of air through upper airway structures; it is an abnormal upper airway sound. Rales (crackles) may indicate disease of the lungs and can be seen with lower airway obstruction. Wheezing is also an abnormal lower airway sound and indicates lower airway obstruction. Rhonchi may be heard in the upper airway but may be normal or abnormal.

Chapter 3: Managing the Pediatric Airway in a Step-by-Step Approach

1. **A.** Begin with positioning the head, suctioning, and providing supplemental oxygen. Your next priority will be to stop the seizure. Endotracheal intubation should NOT be attempted until other maneuvers have been tried and fail. Bag-mask ventilation is not indicated in this patient.

131

Resources

Student Resources

Web Site
www.PediatricAirway.EMSzone.com contains the following student resources to enhance learning and retention of pediatric airway management skills:
- Terminology flashcards
- Online glossary
- Web links

Online Course
The Pediatric Airway Management course is available online at **www.PediatricAirway.EMSzone.com.** Learn the content and practice skills in the safety of a virtual learning environment, at your convenience.

Instructor Resources

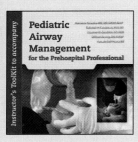

Instructor's ToolKit CD-ROM to accompany Pediatric Airway Management
ISBN: 0-7637-2735-0
This CD includes PowerPoint presentations, lecture outlines, and an image bank containing the figures found in this text.

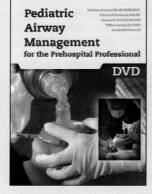

Pediatric Airway Management DVD
ISBN: 0-7637-3284-2
This DVD video shows the ALS and BLS pediatric airway management skills taught in this text. It features real-life field and emergency room footage and stunning animations. Each module opens with a case presentation that continues throughout the module.

Ordering Information
For a complete listing of our EMS products, or to place your order online, please visit **www.EMSzone.com**. To order Jones and Bartlett products by phone, fax, or e-mail, please contact us at:

Jones and Bartlett Publishers
40 Tall Pine Drive
Sudbury, MA 01776
Phone: (978) 443-5000
Fax: (978) 443-8000
info@jbpub.com

Acknowledgments

Jones & Bartlett Publishers and the authors would like to thank the following people for reviewing this text.

Sunil A. Bhopale, MD FACEP
University of California, Davis
School of Medicine
Redwood City, California

Jonnathan M. Busko, MD, MPH, EMT-P
Medical Resource Consulting International
Albany, New York

Terry Crammer, RN, MICN, BSN
Los Angeles County Paramedic Training Institute
Commerce, California

Daniel Doherty, REMT-P
Albany Fire Department
Albany, New York

Steven K. Frye, BS, NREMT-P
University of Maryland
Maryland Fire and Rescue Institute
College Park, Maryland

Jeffrey W. Ongemach, HSC, USCG, AS, NREMT-I
United States Air Force Independent Duty Medical
  Technician School
Sheppard Air Force Base, Texas

Dawn C. Poetter, EMT-P
Metro West Ambulance Training Department
Vernonia, Oregon

Paul E. Sirbaugh, DO, FAAP, FACEP
Baylor College of Medicine
Texas Children's Hospital
Houston, Texas

Charles Stewart, MD, FACEP
Colorado Springs, Colorado

Atilla B. Üner, MD, MPH
UCLA Center for Prehospital Care
Los Angeles, California

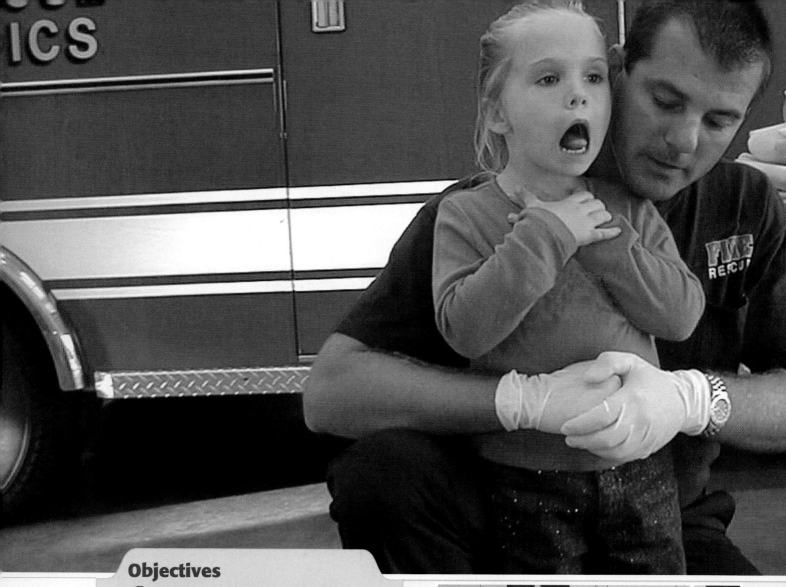

Objectives

1 Identify the important statistics related to respiratory emergencies in children.

2 List four anatomical considerations involved in the airway management of the pediatric patient.

3 Define common terms related to airway emergencies in children.

4 Name two actions necessary to prepare for assessing and treating a child with a respiratory emergency.

5 Describe the role of the prehospital professional in emergency medical services for children.

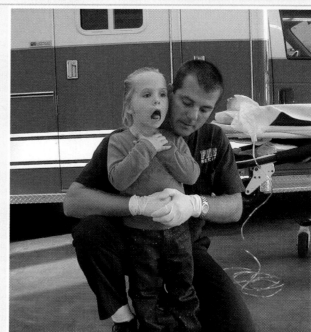

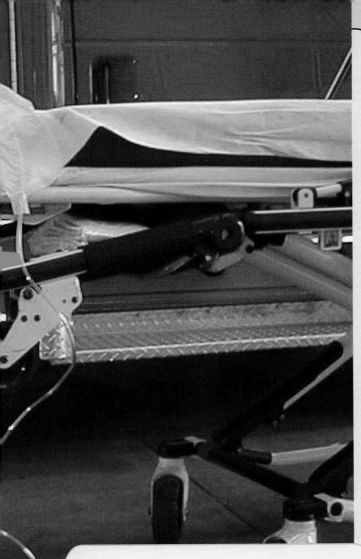

CHAPTER 1

Introduction

Scenario

You are called to the home of a 4-year-old girl with a history of "choking." The mother called 9-1-1 and was given instructions by a dispatcher about how to deliver first aid to her unconscious child; she performed abdominal thrusts without relief of the obstruction.

When you arrive on scene, the patient is unconscious, there is no chest rise, and her skin is cyanotic.

1. *What are your management priorities?*

2. *What anatomical, physiological, and behavioral factors may have led to this child's condition?*

Think about these questions and this case as you read on. We will return to this scenario at the end of the chapter.

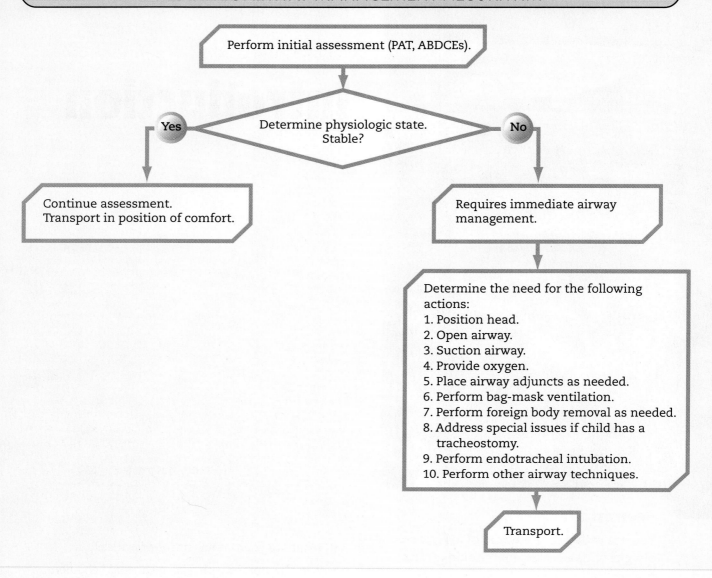

Perform initial assessment (PAT, ABDCEs).

Determine physiologic state. Stable?

Yes → Continue assessment. Transport in position of comfort.

No → Requires immediate airway management.

Determine the need for the following actions:
1. Position head.
2. Open airway.
3. Suction airway.
4. Provide oxygen.
5. Place airway adjuncts as needed.
6. Perform bag-mask ventilation.
7. Perform foreign body removal as needed.
8. Address special issues if child has a tracheostomy.
9. Perform endotracheal intubation.
10. Perform other airway techniques.

Transport.

Who?

Over 30 million children (18 years of age or younger) seek emergency care each year in our nation's emergency departments. Children represent 30% of emergency department patient visits. By contrast, children represent only 10% of all prehospital calls. Of these calls less than 5% are limb- or life-threatening.

The following are definitions of different stages of childhood.

- Neonate: Less than one month of age
- Infant: One month to one year of age
- Child: One year to twelve years of age
- Adolescent: Thirteen years to eighteen years of age

Fifty-seven percent of all pediatric prehospital calls are for traumatic causes, and 43% are for medical complaints. Respiratory complaints comprise 10% of all pediatric prehospital calls; 1% of these patients present in cardiopulmonary arrest from both medical and traumatic causes.

What?

What impact do these statistics have on your practice as a prehospital professional?

- You are less likely to care for a critically ill or injured child than an adult patient; therefore, you have fewer opportunities to gain experience in the care of children.

What can you do to ensure optimal care for your patients?

- Seek out education that includes cognitive (knowledge), affective (attitudes and behaviors), and psychomotor (skills) objectives in the care of children.

- Review and practice assessment and management skills in the care of children.

A multidisciplinary group of emergency professionals has made recommendations about the skills

---

Table 1-1: Essential Skills for Pediatric Education of Paramedics

Assessment of infants and children

Use of a length-based resuscitation tape

Airway management
- Mouth-to-mouth barrier devices
- Oropharyngeal airway
- Nasopharyngeal airway
- Oxygen delivery system
- Bag-mask ventilation
- Endotracheal intubation
- Optional: Endotracheal placement confirmation devices (CO_2 detection), rapid sequence induction
- Foreign body removal with Magill forceps
- Needle thoracostomy
- Nasogastric or orogastric tubes
- Suctioning
- Tracheostomy management

Monitoring
- Cardiorespiratory monitoring
- Pulse oximetry
- End-tidal CO_2 monitoring and/or CO_2 detection

Vascular access
- Intravenous line placement
- Intraosseous line placement

Fluid/medication administration
- Endotracheal
- Intramuscular
- Intravenous
- Nasogastric
- Nebulized
- Oral
- Rectal
- Subcutaneous

Cardioversion

Defibrillation

Drug dosing in infants and children

Immobilization/extrication
- Car seat—extrication
- Spinal immobilization

Adapted from: Gausche M, Henderson DP, Brownstein D, et al. Education of out-of-hospital emergency medical personnel in pediatrics: Report of a national task force. *Ann Emerg Med.* 1998;31:58–63.

---

necessary for the prehospital professional who cares for children. These skills are listed in **Table 1-1**. In addition, this group recommended review of these skills on a regular basis (not to exceed one year).

Where and When?

When assessing a pediatric patient, one of the first decisions you will make as a prehospital provider is whether to manage the patient's medical needs in the field or to initiate rapid transport with advanced management en route to the emergency department. Certainly, patients with respiratory distress or failure will require immediate field management to ensure adequate oxygenation and ventilation en route to the hospital. The question of whether to intubate a patient in the field versus providing bag-mask ventilation is complex and requires knowledge of which intervention is most effective, has the least complications, and promises a better outcome. Although you will always manage the patient's airway immediately, the decision about which techniques should be performed in the field versus the emergency department requires careful consideration, and is likely to change with new research and collective experience.

The Pediatric Airway Management Algorithm presented at the beginning of this chapter shows a methodology for approaching the pediatric patient with a respiratory emergency. This algorithm will be used throughout the text.

Building your knowledge base and applying that knowledge in clinical scenarios can build confidence and reduce the stress of caring for ill and injured children.

Why?

Why is the prehospital airway management of pediatric patients different than that of adult patients?

Predisposing factors for the need for airway management in infants and children are based on anatomical, physiological, and behavioral differences between adults and children.

Anatomical Considerations

video There are numerous anatomical differences in children versus adults relevant to airway management (**Figure 1-1**). Children have:
- A proportionately larger occiput
- A relatively larger tongue
- A larger mass of adenoidal tissues
- An epiglottis that is floppy, long, and more U-shaped

Where's the Evidence?

Frequency of Pediatric Prehospital Care

In a study by Seidel et al of over 10,000 prehospital pediatric calls in 11 California counties, oxygen was given to 23% of pediatric patients and advanced life support skills were rarely used. These data suggest that it would take twenty years for *all* of the paramedics in these counties to perform bag-mask ventilation at least once. Similarly, Glaeser et al found in a survey of over 18,000 EMS providers that 60% of EMT-Paramedics (paramedics), 84% of EMT-Intermediates (EMT-Is), and 87% of EMT-Basics (EMT-Bs) care for less than 3 pediatric patients per month. Seventy-six percent of EMS providers responding to this survey felt that there should be state or national mandates for continuing education in pediatrics.

Gausche, Henderson, and Seidel have shown in a study of over 6,700 pediatric calls in Los Angeles County that assessment of vitals signs varied by age; the younger the child, the less likely the paramedic was to assess all vital signs. Blood pressure was assessed infrequently (12% of the time) in children younger than 3 years of age. Possible reasons for these differences were explored in a survey of over 1,200 paramedics which showed that paramedics were less confident in their ability to take vital signs in younger children. Glaeser et al in a survey performed by the National Registry of EMTs, found that all levels of EMS providers identified infants (1–12 months of age) as the age group of greatest concern when managing a critical patient, and felt that continuing education should be targeted toward this age group. These data suggest that caring for critically ill or injured children can be challenging and stressful.

1. Gausche M. Commentary on the differences in out-of-hospital care of adults and children: More questions than answers. *Ann Emerg Med.* 1997;29:6:776–779.

2. Gausche M, Henderson DP, Seidel JS. Vital signs as a part of the prehospital assessment of the pediatric patient: A survey of paramedics. *Ann Emerg Med.* 1990;19:173–178.

3. Glaeser PW, Linzer J, Tunik MG, et al. Survey of nationally registered emergency medical services providers: Pediatric education. *Ann Emerg Med.* 2000;36:33–74.

4. Seidel JS, Henderson DP, Ward P, et al. Pediatric prehospital care in urban and rural areas. *Pediatrics.* 1991;681–690.

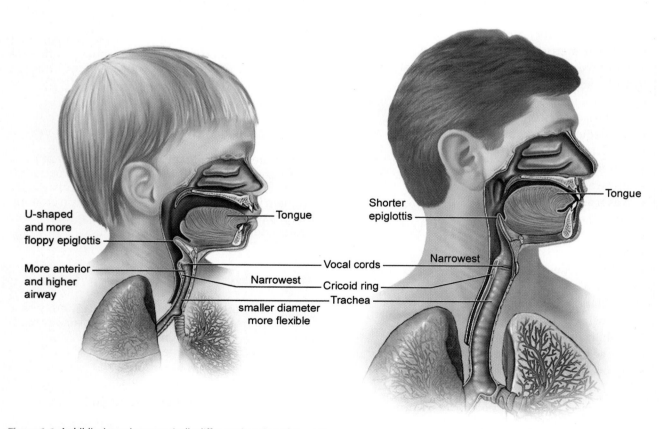

Figure 1-1 A child's airway is anatomically different than that of an adult.

- A <u>larynx</u> (glottis) that is located higher in the neck
- A <u>cricoid ring</u> that is the narrowest portion of the airway
- A narrow <u>tracheal</u> diameter and distance between the rings
- A shorter tracheal length
- Narrower large airways
- A less mature chest and abdominal musculature

Each of these anatomical differences between adults and children can have an impact on the assessment and management of airway and respiratory emergencies.

Larger Occiput

The proportionately larger occiput of the child causes the head to flex on the neck; this can lead to airway obstruction from airway kinking.

- **Actions:** Placement of a small towel under the shoulders of these patients can lift the upper torso, allowing for a level plane of the airway (Figure 1-2).

Larger Tongue

The relatively larger tongue in infants and young children can be a source of airway obstruction, especially in conditions where there is loss of muscle tone (i.e., altered level of consciousness) (Figure 1-3). When performing procedures such as endotracheal intubation, the provider may have more difficulty moving the tongue out of the visual plane of the airway.

- **Actions:** To improve passage of air from the environment to the posterior pharynx, you can reposition the head in the midline, place a towel under the shoulders, or use an airway adjunct (e.g., oropharyngeal [OP] or nasopharyngeal [NP] airway) (Figure 1-4).

Larger Adenoidal Tissues

The presence of a larger mass of adenoidal tissues, especially in infants, can result in greater bleeding com-plications from nasotracheal intubation or placement of a nasopharyngeal airway in infants younger than one year of age.

- **Actions:** Do not perform nasotracheal intubation in infants and young children unless you are experienced in the procedure and it is in the approved scope of practice for your EMS system. Note: VERY FEW providers, including physicians, have great experience in performing this procedure in children.
- Use other airway opening techniques (e.g., head tilt-chin lift) before nasopharyngeal airway placement to keep the airway open. If none of these are successful, then placement of a nasopharyngeal airway is an option.

Floppy, Long, U-shaped Epiglottis

The epiglottis in a child is floppy, long, and more U-shaped than in an adult (Figure 1-5), making visualization of the <u>vocal cords</u> difficult. The configuration of the epiglottis of a child becomes more like an adult's after 3 years of age.

- **Actions:** May necessitate use of a straight blade in children to lift the epiglottis directly out of the visual plane of the airway.

Higher Larynx

The larynx (glottis) is higher and more forward in the neck (glottis at C3-4 in newborns, C4-5 by 2 years of age, and C5-6 in adults) thus making it more difficult for the provider to visualize the vocal cords with the child on the floor or at ground level (Figure 1-6).

- **Actions:** Elevate the patient on a gurney or table or place yourself lower than the patient and look up, at a 45-degree angle or greater, to visualize the airway when performing advanced life support (e.g., foreign body removal with Magill forceps or intubation). Cricoid pressure (mild) may be necessary to see the glottic opening.

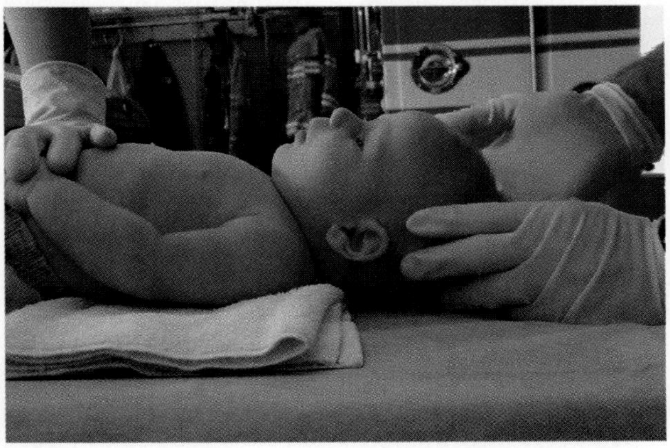

Figure 1-2 Place a small towel under a child's shoulders to prevent airway obstruction.

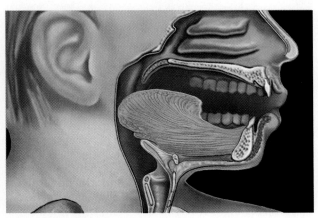

Figure 1-3 The relatively larger tongue of a child can obstruct the airway when there is loss of muscle tone.

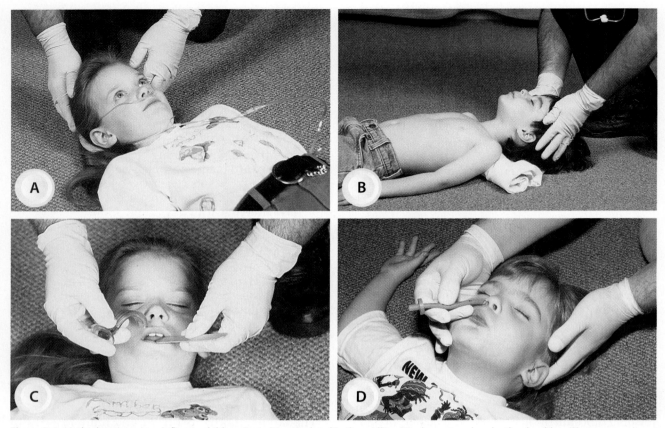

Figure 1-4 Methods to improve air flow in children: Reposition the head in the midline (A), place a towel under the shoulders (B), or use an airway adjunct such as an oropharyngeal (C) or nasopharyngeal airway (D).

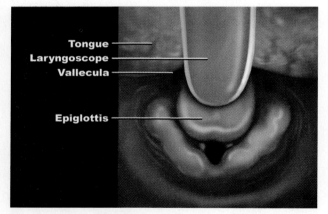

Figure 1-5 A child's epiglottis is floppier, longer, and more U-shaped than an adult's.

Figure 1-6 The larynx is positioned higher and more forward in the neck in children.

Narrower Cricoid Ring

The cricoid ring is the narrowest portion of the airway up to age 5 years; after this age the narrowest point is at the glottis (Figure 1-7).

- **Actions:** Uncuffed tubes are used in infants and in children up to size 6.0 mm endotracheal tube or about 8 years of age. An inflated endotracheal cuff pushing firmly on the cricoid ring could cause enough pressure to limit the blood supply

to this cartilaginous ring, causing it to deteriorate. Cuffed endotracheal tubes are used in certain critically ill or injured patients in intensive care settings when high pressures are required to ventilate the patient—the cuff in this situation is closely monitored to prevent damage to the cricoid ring. In emergency care settings, it is best to begin with an uncuffed tube in children receiving a size 5.5 mm or less endotracheal tube.

Narrower Tracheal Diameter

The narrow tracheal diameter and shorter distance between the rings makes performing a tracheostomy more difficult in infants and young children.

- **Actions:** Consider needle cricothyrotomy for the difficult airway in children if the airway cannot be maintained with bag-mask ventilation *and* endotracheal intubation. See Chapter 8 for coverage of this procedure.

Shorter Tracheal Length

The shorter length of the trachea in children (4–5 cm in newborn; 7–8 cm in 18 month old) (Figure 1-8) can lead to intubation of the right mainstem bronchus or dislodgement of the endotracheal tube.

- **Actions:** Use the length-based resuscitation (Broselow) tape to determine endotracheal tube

size and depth of tube placement (Figure 1-9). While performing endotracheal intubation, place the vocal cord marker (if present) on the endotracheal tube just below the vocal cords; there is no need to insert the tube deeper into the airway. As a general rule, depth of endotracheal tube placement at the lip (in centimeters) can be estimated by multiplying three times the internal diameter of the endotracheal tube. These steps will help to prevent mainstem intubation.

- Reassess the intubated patient for endotracheal tube position whenever the patient is moved, as dislodgement may easily occur.
- Immobilize the patient to prevent head movement.

Narrower Airway

The airway of the child is narrower (Figure 1-10), resulting in greater airway resistance; resistance is proportional

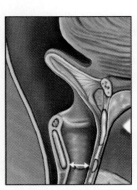 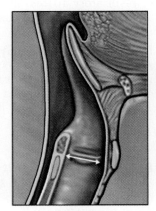

Narrowest portion of pediatric airway = cricoid

Narrowest portion of adult airway = vocal cords

Figure 1-7 The narrowest portion of the pediatric airway is at the cricoid ring.

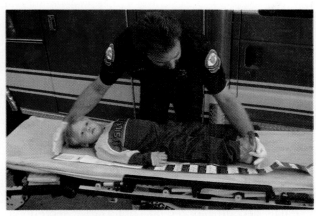

Figure 1-9 Use the length-based resuscitation tape to determine endotracheal tube size and depth of tube placement.

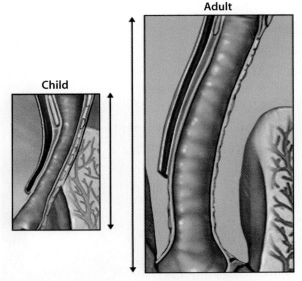

Figure 1-8 The trachea is shorter in children than in adults.

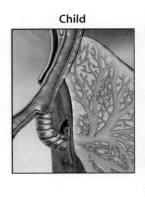 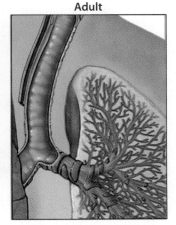

Figure 1-10 A child's airway is narrow than an adult's. This results in greater resistance.

to 1/radius⁴. This means that as the radius of a child's airway is reduced by half, the resistance increases 16 times.

- **Actions:** Suction all patients liberally, particularly if they are producing large amounts of secretions, as secretions can easily cause increased airway resistance or obstruction. This is especially important in a patient with a tracheostomy because the insertion of the tracheostomy tube further narrows the airway, and the lumen can easily become blocked by a build-up of secretions on the inner walls.

Less Mature Chest and Abdominal Musculature

The less mature chest and abdominal musculature of the child results in easy fatigue of the diaphragm.

- **Actions:** Begin assisted ventilation with bag-mask ventilation in children with poor tidal volume (chest rise) and signs of respiratory failure.

Physiological and Behavioral Considerations

video Physiological and behavioral differences in children versus adults relevant to airway management include:

- Preferential nose breathing for the first several months of life
- Higher metabolic requirements
- Inefficient immune system in small infants
- Behavioral immaturity (unable to verbalize distress)

Each of these physiological or behavioral differences in adults and children can have an impact on the assessment and management of airway and respiratory emergencies.

Preferential Nose Breathing

Preferential nose breathing results in respiratory distress if the nasal passages are blocked.

- **Actions:** Suction the nose and mouth of infants to remove mucus, blood, or meconium. This action may relieve the respiratory distress.

Higher Metabolic Requirements

Higher metabolic requirements increase the need for oxygen and nutrients, resulting in higher normal respiratory rates in infants and children.

- **Actions:** Supply oxygen to all children in respiratory distress and know normal respiratory rates in infants and children (Figure 1-11).

Inefficient Immune System

An inefficient immune system in small infants results in a greater likelihood for respiratory infections.

- **Actions:** Assess infants and children with fever, respiratory distress or failure, or with altered level of consciousness for respiratory disease including infection.

Behavioral Immaturity

Behavioral immaturity results in the infant or young child's inability to verbalize respiratory distress or communicate clues as to its cause.

- **Actions:** Practice assessment skills on all ages of children so that you are able to distinguish stable children from those in respiratory distress or failure.

Definitions

video The following are terms that you will see throughout this text. They are presented here

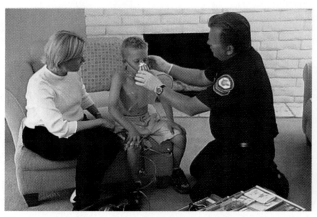

Figure 1-11 Supply oxygen to children in respiratory distress.

to help you become familiar with topics you will be studying.

- Respiratory distress: A condition characterized by increased work of breathing.
- Respiratory failure: A condition in which compensatory mechanisms are no longer able to maintain adequate oxygenation or ventilation.
- Respiratory arrest: A condition defined by absence of spontaneous respiration.
- Upper airway obstruction: Obstruction of airflow from the level of the oropharynx to the mainstem bronchi.
- Lower airway obstruction: Obstruction of airflow from the mainstem bronchi to the end of the smallest air passages (bronchioles).
- Disease of the lungs: A condition that prevents adequate gas-exchange in the lung; this may be caused by the presence of fluid (edema or pus) or collapse or destruction of the air sacs (alveoli).

■ Preparation for Airway and Respiratory Emergencies

Preparation for managing airway and respiratory emergencies in children can occur at a number of levels. These levels include federal, state, regional, local, and individual.

The EMS for Children (EMSC) Program is a national initiative administered by the Health Resources and Services Administration's (HRSA), Maternal and Child Health Bureau (MCHB), and the Department of Transportation's National Highway Traffic Safety Administration (NHTSA). EMSC was established in 1985 to help reduce childhood disability and death due to severe illness or injury. EMSC promotes integration of pediatric components into EMS systems. Aspects of EMSC include injury and illness prevention, access to care (9-1-1), prehospital care, emergency department care, hospital care, and rehabilitation. EMSC components may be integrated into your EMS system to a greater or lesser degree.

Your Role in EMSC

You can participate in improving EMSC by advocating for improvements in education and training, prevention programs, patient care protocols, system policies, and legislation at federal, state, and local levels (Figure 1-12). Individually, you can prepare your station and service for a critical child emergency by:

- Ensuring that you have available the appropriate-sized equipment and supplies (Figure 1-13)
- Obtaining the knowledge of pediatric emergency care necessary to assess and treat an infant, child, or adolescent; and
- Practicing pediatric airway management skills to maintain a high level of proficiency in the care of critically ill or injured pediatric patients.

Actions

What are your immediate actions when you get a call such as the one presented in the beginning of this chapter?

- Before all calls, you should check your pediatric equipment, including:
  - Airway equipment in sizes for pediatric patients
  - Length-based resuscitation tape, or other means of weight estimation
  - Chart or reference with age-related dosages of medications
  - Seat restraints, child car seat
- Once dispatched, you should obtain information about the child, including:
  - Age
  - Gender
  - Chief complaint/mechanism of injury
  - Cultural issues (Does the child or parent[s] speak a foreign language?)
  - Special needs (Remember to obtain information on baseline status of the patient.)
- En route, you should:
  - Review team roles
  - Review possible management priorities

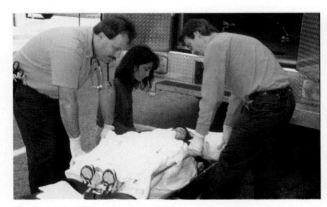

Figure 1-12 EMS plays a vital role in the welfare of children.

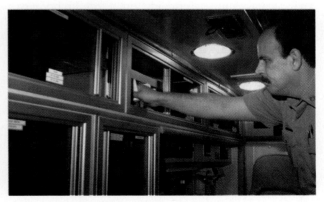

Figure 1-13 Ensure that you have the appropriate-sized pediatric equipment and supplies.

Conclusions

EMS providers have few opportunities to care for critically ill or injured children; therefore pediatric emergency education is a crucial component of prehospital practice. Understanding the airway differences between children and adults and the definitions important to the assessment and management of a child with a respiratory emergency are the first steps in this education. EMS providers play a vital role in the welfare of our nation's children as advocates for EMSC.

Scenario Review

You were called to the home of a 4-year-old girl with a history of "choking." The mother had called 9-1-1 and a dispatcher had given her instructions for administering first aid to her unconscious child. She performed abdominal thrusts without relief of the obstruction. When you arrived at the house, the patient was unconscious, there was no chest rise, and the child's skin was cyanotic.

1. *What are your management priorities?*

The first step in management is assessment. Chapter 2 will outline the steps required to properly assess the pediatric patient. Your assessment of this patient shows abnormal appearance, absent work of breathing, and signs of impaired circulation, all of which indicate respiratory or cardiopulmonary failure. You immediately begin assisted ventilation with 100% oxygen by bag-mask ventilation and continue your assessment. You find the patient does not have a pulse, so CPR is initiated and a monitor is placed which shows bradycardia at a rate of 40 beats per minute.

Let's stop here. There is much more to discuss with this case but we will do so in subsequent chapters.

2. *What anatomical, physiological, and behavioral factors may have led to this child's condition?*

Children under the age of 5 are most likely to aspirate a foreign body because of their insatiable curiosity. Young children explore by putting objects in their mouths. The small size of the child's airway places him or her at increased risk for complete airway obstruction. Because the narrowest portion of the pediatric airway is at the cricoid ring, a foreign body can be lodged below the level of the cords, making removal of the object particularly difficult. Also, the flexible tracheal rings can be compressed by a large esophageal foreign body. The prominent occiput in this child will necessitate great care in positioning the airway for optimal airway opening. The immature chest and abdominal muscles are less likely to assist in expelling the foreign body by coughing.

Quick Quiz

1. *Children represent, on average, what percentage of all prehospital calls?*
   - A. 10%
   - B. 25%
   - C. 40%
   - D. 50%

2. *Which of the following correctly identifies airway differences in children versus adults?*
   - A. The epiglottis is floppy and U-shaped, the occiput is prominent, the cricoid is the narrowest portion of the airway.
   - B. The airway is larger, the tracheal rings are stiffer, the vocal cords are c-shaped.
   - C. The tongue is relatively large, the abdominal and chest musculature is more developed, the trachea is longer.
   - D. The distance between the tracheal rings is smaller, children have a slower metabolic rate, the larynx is lower in the neck.

3. *What action can you take to prevent or treat respiratory distress that may result from the fact that young infants are preferential nose breathers?*
   - A. Place a towel under the shoulders.
   - B. Place a nasopharyngeal airway.
   - C. Suction the nose to remove secretions.
   - D. Use a nasal cannula to supply supplemental oxygen.

4. *What is your role in Emergency Medical Services for Children (EMSC)?*
   - A. Advocate for children to ensure that your EMS system is prepared to care for children and prevent injury.
   - B. Ensure that your station has the equipment to care for children.
   - C. Maintain your knowledge and skills in the care of children.
   - D. All of the above

5. *Which of the following statements defines respiratory distress?*
   - A. Absence of breathing
   - B. Poor tidal volume
   - C. Cyanosis
   - D. Increased work of breathing

Glossary

adenoidal tissue   Lymphoid tissue in the back of the mouth and oropharynx.

cricoid ring   A ring of cartilage that encircles the larynx.

disease of the lungs   A condition that prevents adequate gas-exchange in the lung; this may be caused by the presence of fluid (edema or pus) or collapse or destruction of the air sacs (alveoli).

epiglottis   A thin, leaf-shaped structure located immediately posterior to the root of the tongue that prevents food and secretions from entering the trachea.

larynx   The enlarged upper end of the trachea, below the root of the tongue, that contains the vocal cords.

lower airway obstruction   Obstruction of airflow from the mainstem bronchi to the end of the smallest air passages (bronchioles).

meconium   The thick, sticky, dark green first stools of the newborn.

occiput   The back part of the skull.

respiratory arrest   A condition defined by absence of spontaneous respiration.

respiratory distress   A condition characterized by increased work of breathing.

respiratory failure   A condition where compensatory mechanisms are no longer able to maintain adequate oxygenation or ventilation.

trachea   A cylindrical cartilaginous tube from the larynx to the bronchial tubes. It extends from the 6th cervical to the 5th dorsal vertebra, where it divides at a point called the carina into two bronchi, one leading to each lung.

upper airway obstruction   Obstruction of airflow from the level of the oropharynx to the mainstem bronchi.

vocal cords   Either of two pairs of folds of mucous membrane of which each member contains a band of fibrous tissue and a free edge projecting into the larynx.

Selected References

1. Baren JM, Seidel JSS. Emergency Management of Respiratory Distress and Failure. In: Barkin RM (ed) *Pediatric Emergency Medicine: Concepts and Clinical Practice,* Mosby-Yearbook, St. Louis,1997; 95–103.

2. Dieckmann RA, Brownstein D, Gausche-Hill M (eds). *Pediatric Education for Prehospital Professionals: PEPP Textbook,* Jones & Bartlett Publishers, Sudbury, MA, 2000;58–77.

3. Gausche-Hill M, Dieckmann RA, Brownstein D (eds). *Pediatric Education for Prehospital Professionals: PEPP Resource Manual,* Jones & Bartlett Publishers, Sudbury, MA, 2000;60–71.

4. Gausche M. Commentary on the differences in out-of-hospital care of adults and children: More questions than answers. *Ann Emerg Med.* 1997;29:6:776–779.

5. Gausche M, Henderson DP, Brownstein D, et al. Education of out-of-hospital emergency medical personnel in pediatrics: Report of a national task force. *Ann Emerg Med.* 1998;31:58–63.

6. Gausche M, Henderson DP, Seidel JS. Vital signs as a part of the prehospital assessment of the pediatric patient: A survey of paramedics. *Ann Emerg Med.* 1990;19:173–178.

7. Gausche M, Lewis RJ, Stratton SJ, et al. Effect of out-of-hospital pediatric endotracheal intubation on survival and neurological outcome: A controlled clinical trial. *JAMA.* 2000;283:6:783–790.

8. Glaeser PW, Linzer J, Tunik MG, et al. Survey of nationally registered emergency medical services providers: Pediatric education. *Ann Emerg Med.* 2000;36:33–74.

9. Seidel JS, Henderson DP, Ward P, et al. Pediatric prehospital care in urban and rural areas. *Pediatrics.* 1991;681–690.

10. Tsai A, Kallsen G. Epidemiology of pediatric prehospital care. *Ann Emerg Med.* 1987;16:284–292.

End of Chapter Activities

Technology Resources

Online Course

Anatomy Review

Online Glossary

Web Links

Online Quiz

Scenarios

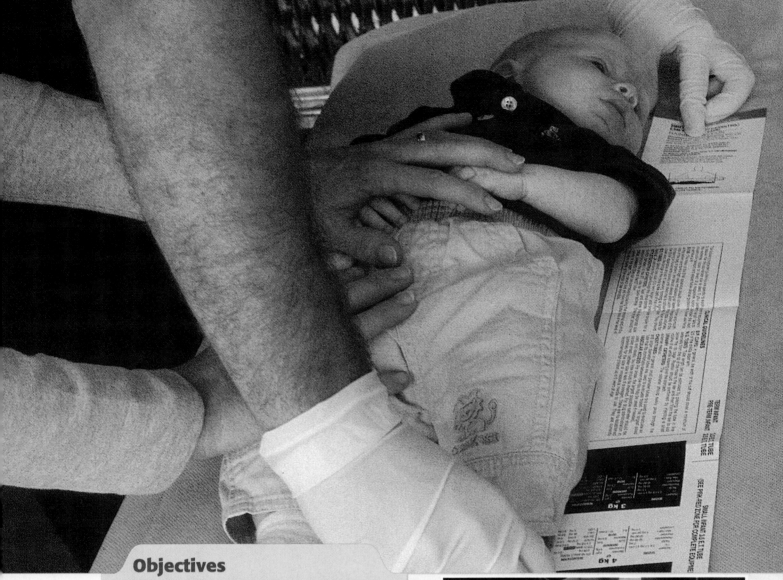

Objectives

1 Describe the systematic method of assessing a child, from initial contact through secondary assessment.

2 Assess the severity of respiratory distress and failure by using the initial assessment sequence.

3 Differentiate the categories of respiratory dysfunction by using the initial assessment sequence.

4 Outline priorities in airway management based on the initial and secondary impressions.

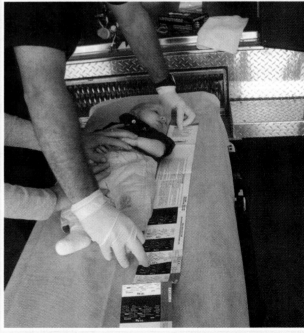

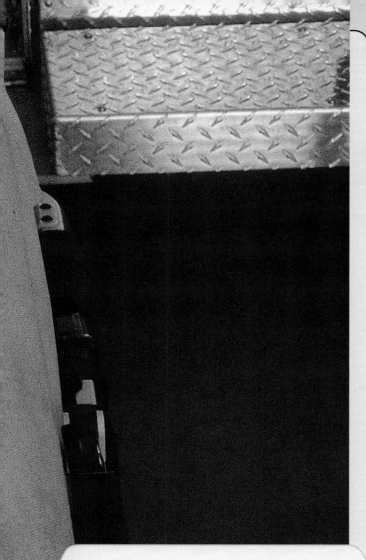

CHAPTER 2

Assessment

Scenario

You receive a call to go to a park where you find a 2-year-old girl whose mother says the child is having difficulty breathing.

1. *How would you begin your assessment?*

2. *How do you determine the seriousness of the patient's condition?*

Think about these questions and this case as you read on. We will return to this scenario at the end of the chapter.

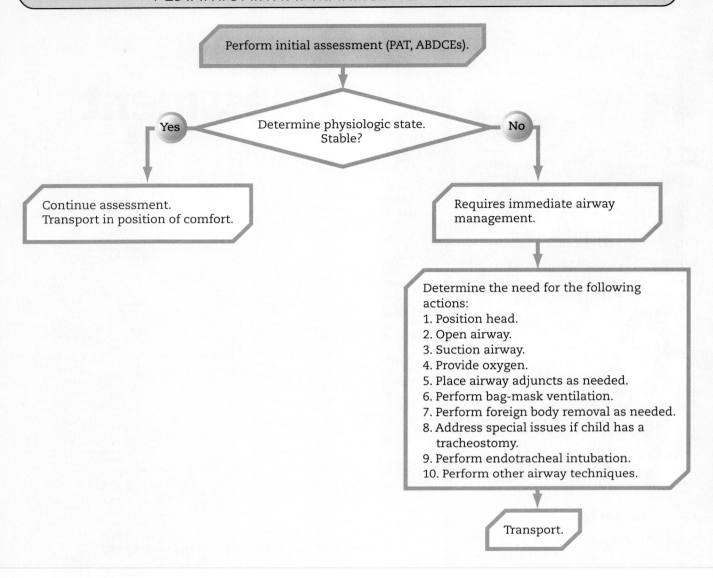

Perform initial assessment (PAT, ABDCEs).

Determine physiologic state. Stable?

Yes → Continue assessment. Transport in position of comfort.

No → Requires immediate airway management.

Determine the need for the following actions:
1. Position head.
2. Open airway.
3. Suction airway.
4. Provide oxygen.
5. Place airway adjuncts as needed.
6. Perform bag-mask ventilation.
7. Perform foreign body removal as needed.
8. Address special issues if child has a tracheostomy.
9. Perform endotracheal intubation.
10. Perform other airway techniques.

Transport.

Introduction

Careful assessment is the key to recognizing injury and illness in all patients. Because children have less experience with illness and may be less articulate than adults and, in some cases, preverbal (have not yet developed speech), assessing the pediatric patient requires an even more systematic and observant approach. When you follow a consistent pattern of assessment, you can be sure that nothing is overlooked and that subsequent treatment is appropriate and tailored to the specific needs of the child. There are two components to initial prehospital assessment of the pediatric patient:

1. Pediatric Assessment Triangle (PAT)

2. ABCDEs

Careful assessment will lead to your decision about the need for immediate treatment and the method and speed of transport necessary for the patient.

The Pediatric Assessment Triangle

The purpose of the Pediatric Assessment Triangle (PAT) is to obtain an immediate general impression of the seriousness of the illness or injury. The focus is on visual and auditory clues about 1) general appearance; 2) work of breathing; and 3) circulatory status of the infant or child (Figure 2-1).

General Appearance

Assessment of the general appearance includes observation of certain characteristics (Figure 2-2). To remember these, you can use the TICLS mnemonic:

T: Tone (muscle): Observe how the child reacts when you begin your examination. Does she lie there quietly, or resist? Does she seem weak or listless?

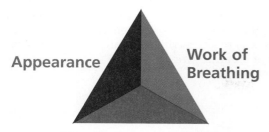

Figure 2-1 The three components of the Pediatric Assessment Triangle include Appearance, Work of Breathing, and Circulation to the Skin.

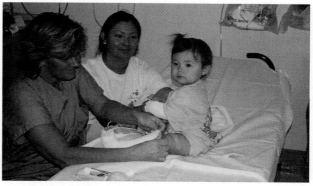

Figure 2-2 Appearance shows the patient with normal tone, interactiveness, and normal look/gaze for age.

I: Interactiveness: How alert is the child? Is there resistance to your examination? Do moving or shiny objects catch her eye and does she follow movements? Is the child playful and interactive?

C: Consolability: When the child is crying, can she be consoled by her mother or other caregiver? Is her crying unrelieved by distraction or other measures?

L: Look/Gaze: Do her eyes seem to focus on objects and look directly at other people, or is her gaze fixed and unfocused?

S: Speech/Cry: Is her crying loud and strong, or does it seem to be weak or hoarse?

When you assess the general appearance, you develop an overall impression ("snapshot") of how sick the child is at that moment. The general impression includes attention to:

- The child's developmental age, and
- The child's physical development.

A 9-month-old infant, for instance, may be afraid of strangers, avoid your eyes, and cry when examined. This would be a normal response for that child's age. Some general descriptions of developmental levels of children and possible interventions are included in **Table 2-1**.

Table 2-1: Child Development Issues

	Developmental Stage	Perceptions	Interventions
Birth to 18 mos.	Egocentric Learning to trust	Mainly physical perceptions—warmth, hunger, being held	Keep warm. Keep with caregiver. Allow pacifier or bottle if appropriate.
18 mos. to 3 yrs.	Learning independence Walking Toilet training	Dislikes being restrained Lives in the here and now	Avoid restraint as much as possible. Allow caregiver to comfort during procedures.
3 to 6 yrs.	Beginning to talk, communicate Prelogical thinking	Magical thinking May see pain as punishment Fantasizes about fears	Be honest. Inform of procedures. Give praise regardless of behavior.
6 to 12 yrs.	Logical, concrete thinking Begins school	Begins to understand causality Learns fear of death	Explain procedures. Enlist cooperation. Give choices. Distract with games, counting. Give rewards, praise.
12 to 18 yrs.	Abstract thinking, Developing self-image	Easily embarrassed Understands emotional vs. physical pain	Fully explain procedures. Encourage questions. Allow participation. Avoid teasing. Maintain modesty.

A child is probably not critically ill or injured if he/she:
- Is alert
- Watches you as you approach
- Responds interactively
- Has good color

However, the potential for serious illness still exists—a child who appears initially normal may, for example, have an epidural hematoma or may have ingested a toxic substance and could become seriously ill in the very near future. These possibilities will have to be explored during the full assessment and evaluation process.

Work of Breathing

Assessment of the work of breathing gives you an idea of the oxygenation and ventilation of the child. Oxygenation refers to how well tissues are getting oxygen, while ventilation refers to how well air is being moved in and out of the lungs. Respiratory rates vary by age and can be affected by a wide variety of factors, so the work of breathing is often a more rapid and accurate way to assess the respiratory status of a child. Work of breathing includes:
- Airway sounds
- Positioning
- Use of accessory muscles

Airway Sounds

The normal swishing of air in and out through the trachea can rarely be heard at a distance, although the sounds are audible with a stethoscope. Many *abnormal* airway sounds are easily audible without a stethoscope. Abnormal airway sounds indicate obstruction to the passage of air through the airway structures. The type of abnormal airway sound is related to whether the disease is in the upper airway, as with gurgling or stridor, or in the lower airways such as the alveoli, bronchioles, and bronchi, as with rales (crackles) or wheezing (Figure 2-3). A brief description of the sounds and their causes is shown in **Table 2-2**.

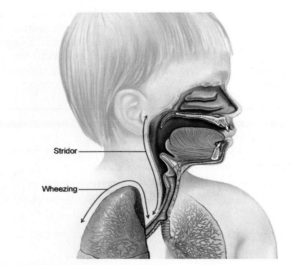

Figure 2-3 Anatomical location of various abnormal airway sounds.

Positioning

Children instinctively position themselves to maximize the opening of the airway when there is airway obstruction, regardless of cause. A child will assume the "sniffing position" (nose held up, head flexed back) to improve the flow of air by lining up the axes of the airway. If the child is old enough to sit up (usually over six months of age), she will do so, and may lean forward, resting on her outstretched hands (tripod position) to maximize airway opening (Figure 2-4). Both of these positions are good indicators of respiratory distress and possible partial airway obstruction.

Accessory Muscle Use

In quiet breathing, the main muscle of respiration is the diaphragm. Contraction of the diaphragm lowers pressure in the thoracic cavity drawing air into the lungs. Expiration is a passive act, caused by relaxation of the respiratory muscles and the elastic contraction of the chest wall. When there is an additional oxygen demand, other muscles are used to aid in breathing. For example, the intercostal muscles raise the ribs up and out, increasing the volume of the thoracic cavity. Other muscles, such as the muscles of the abdominal wall, are used to assist in active exhalation. Use of accessory muscles for normal breathing causes retractions, which are therefore good indicators of respiratory distress.

Retractions can be seen in several areas of the chest:
- Supraclavicular area (above the clavicles)
- Intercostal area (between the ribs)
- Substernal area (under the sternum), depending on the muscles used to aid in respiration (Figure 2-5).

There are two other indicators of accessory muscle use and respiratory distress:
- Head bobbing
- Nasal flaring

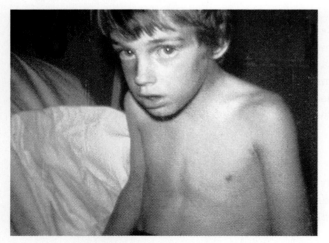

Figure 2-4 Tripod position to open the airway in a child with upper airway obstruction (epiglottitis).

Table 2-2: Abnormal Airway Sounds

Airway Sound	Description	Location	Possible Cause	Intervention
Gurgling	Gurgling, bubbling noise	Posterior pharynx Upper airway	Uncleared secretions or fluid in pharynx or upper larynx	Oxygen Suction
Rhonchi	Low pitched musical, rough, rattling sound	Upper airway Mainstem bronchus	Secretions, fluids, or narrowing in the larger airways	Oxygen Observe for adequate ventilation and oxygenation Suction
Grunting	Brief, pressured vocalization on expiration due to a partially closed glottis	Upper airway	Instinctive creation of partial occlusion in the upper airway, resulting in positive end expiratory pressure (PEEP)	Oxygen Support of ventilation as needed
Stridor	High pitched crowing or barking sound usually heard on inspiration. May also be heard on both expiration and inspiration.	Upper airway	Air passing through narrowed laryngeal or sublottic airway; may be foreign body obstruction, croup, epiglottitis, or an allergic reaction	Oxygen Allow patient to assume position of comfort Support ventilation for patients in respiratory failure Rapid transport
Wheezing	Whistling, musical sound present on expiration or inspiration	Lower airways: bronchioles, alveoli	Usually airway disease Partially obstructed lower airways Asthma is most common cause	Oxygen May assist with inhaler or provide nebulized albuterol Airway management if appropriate
Absence of sound (conscious patient)	No sound on auscultation	Complete airway obstruction	Obstructed airway due to foreign body or airway disease	Oxygen Obtain history Airway management for presumed cause Rapid transport
Rales (Crackles)	Fine, high- to medium-pitched crackling sounds heard mid to late inspiration	Air sacs (alveoli)	Fluid/mucus in air sacs Lower airway disease: pneumonia is most common cause	Oxygen Observe for adequate ventilation and oxygenation

Head bobbing is caused by extension (tilting backwards) of the head on the neck in an effort to open the airway; the head then relaxes forward on exhalation. Nasal flaring (opening of the nostrils to their widest point) also allows passage of more air and is an indication of moderate to severe respiratory distress (Figure 2-6).

When there is any difficulty breathing, the infant or child uses these compensatory mechanisms to assist in oxygenation and ventilation. In addition, look for an anxious expression on the child's face. Early airway obstruction in any form causes extreme anxiety.

To evaluate a patient's work of breathing from across the room:

- Observe for signs of anxiety.
- Note any abnormal breathing sounds.
- Look at the way she is positioned.

- Determine if she is using accessory muscles for respiration.

This quick assessment gives you a sense of the respiratory status of the child.

Circulation to the Skin

The third component of the Pediatric Assessment Triangle is circulatory status. Although circulatory assessment often includes counting the heart rate, at this point, it is not necessary to count the beats. More importantly, observe the skin. When there is inadequate blood volume in the circulatory system or when the heart is unable to maintain output to the body, blood supply to vital organs is conserved by shutting down circulation to the less essential areas of the body, such as the skin and mucous membranes. The signs of inadequate perfusion (blood flow to tissues) include:

- Pallor (paleness)
- Cyanosis (bluish color) of the skin and mucous membranes.
- Mottling (bluish purple patchy irregular areas) of the skin. This is caused by uneven constriction of capillary beds in the skin (Figure 2-7).

In infants less than 2 months of age acrocyanosis (bluish color of the hands and feet) may be present as a normal finding—it simply reflects vasomotor (ability of the blood vessels to dilate or contract) instability of the infant.

To assess circulation to the child's skin:

- Observe any exposed skin on the face and extremities.
- Skin color can be affected by cool environmental temperature, so take into consideration the temperature of the room.
- Ask the caregiver to partially undress the child (being careful to maintain modesty, especially in older children) and observe the chest and abdomen.
- Look at the skin and mucous membranes for signs of pallor or cyanosis. It may be more difficult to assess pallor and mottling in children with dark skin, so carefully observe the mucous membranes of the mouth and pull the lower eyelid down to look at the conjunctival membranes.

These three assessments, General Appearance, Work of Breathing, and Circulatory Status, form the Pediatric Assessment Triangle (PAT). These give a rapid overall impression of whether the child's illness or injury is severe and life-threatening, before you perform a more thorough evaluation and a hands-on examination. The PAT helps determine how rapidly you need to intervene and what additional assistance or treatments may be needed immediately.

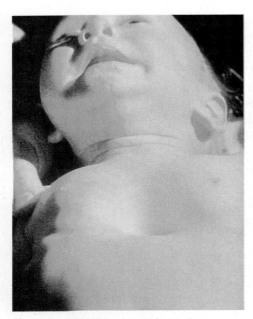

Figure 2-5 Child with substernal retractions.

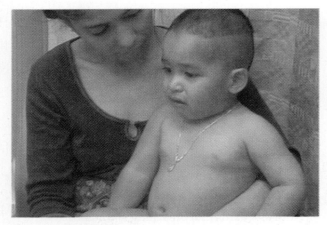

Figure 2-6 Nasal flaring.

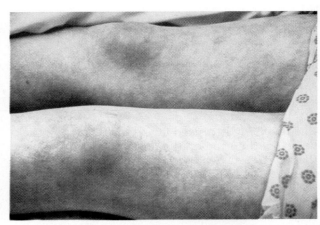

Figure 2-7 Mottling of the skin which represents capillary beds clamping down in response to poor perfusion.

The ABCDEs

The second part of your overall assessment includes physical assessment of the ABCDEs, similar to the process for adults: Airway, Breathing, Circulation, Disability, and Exposure. After assessment of the PAT and ABCDEs, you should have a clear picture of whether the patient is stable or unstable.

Airway

In the PAT, you determined whether there was any degree of difficulty breathing or airway obstruction and where that obstruction might be. As you observe more carefully, make sure that the chest is rising adequately. If there appears to be upper airway obstruction, check whether there is a foreign body in the mouth or in the back of the throat.

Breathing

Assess the child's breathing by determining how fast or slow the child is breathing and by listening to the child's chest (Figure 2-8).

Additional information about respiratory status can be obtained with pulse oximetry, although any interpretation of pulse oximetry readings should be combined with assessment of respiratory rate, work of breathing, and chest auscultation to obtain an accurate picture of respiratory status.

Respiratory Rate

Exercise, emotion, temperature, and other factors may increase a child's respiratory rate, but a respiratory rate that is very high with increased work of breathing is a danger sign. Observe the child and note whether the breathing seems abnormally fast or slow.

Auscultation

Listening to the child's chest can provide valuable information. Whether or not abnormal breath sounds are heard in the PAT assessment, abnormal sounds such as crackles, wheezing, stridor, and grunting can be assessed with a stethoscope and sometimes may be audible even without a stethoscope (Table 2-2). Be aware that loud upper airway sounds often are transmitted when listening to the lungs, and thus those upper airways sounds may sound as if they are coming from the lungs.

Pulse Oximetry

If pulse oximetry equipment is available, it can serve as a useful adjunct to other assessments (Figure 2-9). Remember, however, that pulse oximetry only measures oxygen saturation of the blood cells, so an anemic child, or a child who has lost a significant amount of blood, for instance, may have adequate oxygen saturation, but insufficient oxygenation. Pulse oximetry readings should always be evaluated alongside other assessments, especially work of breathing.

Circulation

After obtaining a general impression of circulatory status from looking at the circulation to the skin in the PAT, make a more in-depth assessment by measuring the rate and quality of the child's pulse, checking the skin temperature, assessing capillary refill time, and taking the child's blood pressure.

Rate and Quality of Pulse

A very rapid pulse can be an indicator of hypoxia, blood loss, and impending shock. There can also be many common and non–life-threatening causes of increased heart rate including anxiety, pain, body temperature, excitement, and exercise. Serial assessments may help in determining the cause and seriousness of a rapid heart rate. If the heart rate increases significantly in a short period, and the child seems ill, hypoxia or shock may be the cause. If an ill or injured child initially has a rapid heart rate and it slows to bradycardia (slow heart rate), the child may be going into shock, respi-

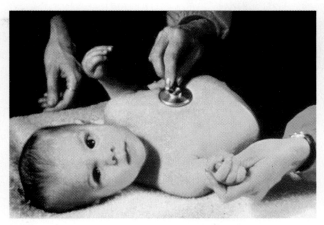

Figure 2-8 Listen to the child's chest to assess breath sounds.

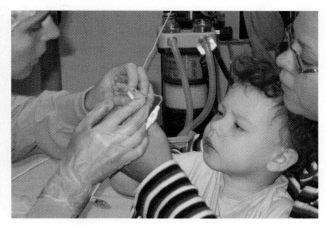

Figure 2-9 Placing a pulse oximeter probe on a toddler.

ratory failure, or cardiopulmonary failure. Bradycardia is a late sign of cardiovascular collapse.

Skin Temperature

Consider the environmental temperature when you assess the skin temperature of a child. With their smaller bodies, children are very susceptible to changes in temperature. In a warm room, the child's extremities should be warm to the touch. Lack of perfusion may cause cool skin; the cooling moves from the distal extremities centrally toward the heart. If lack of perfusion is a concern, evaluate skin temperature along with other signs of shock.

Capillary Refill Time

Capillary refill time can give some indication of circulatory status. Assess capillary refill time as follows:

- Choose an area such as the kneecap, forearm, toe, or finger, where you can press skin against bone.
- Ensure that the chosen area for assessing capillary refill is at the level of the heart or above. Sometimes choosing an area below the level of the heart can lead to a false sense of normal perfusion.
- Press the child's skin against the bony area and release, while counting the seconds until the area is reperfused (becomes normal color again) (Figure 2-10).
- Greater than two to three seconds for reperfusion can indicate inadequate circulation.

Although the importance of this assessment is controversial, capillary refill is still a useful tool. Room temperature and other factors have been shown to affect capillary refill time.

Blood Pressure

It is usually not helpful to obtain the infant or child's blood pressure during the early part of assessment. A child in shock can have a normal, increased, or decreased blood pressure. In addition, blood pressures

Where's the Evidence?

Capillary Refill Time

Two studies have shown that several factors affect capillary refill time. One study by Schriger and Baraff showed that capillary refill was dependent on age and temperature in adults, children, and elderly patients. Immersion in cold water significantly increased capillary refill time in all patients. This study noted that capillary refill time should be considered an unreliable assessment in the prehospital setting. Gorelick, Shaw, and Baker assessed capillary refill time of children at different ambient temperatures, and found that there was significant prolongation of capillary refill time in cool temperature, even in children with normal circulatory status. These studies indicate that variations in ambient temperature should be taken into consideration when capillary refill time is assessed.

1. Gorelick MH, Shaw KN, Baker MD. Effect of ambient temperature on capillary refill in healthy children. *Pediatrics*. 1993;92(5):699–702.
2. Schriger DL, Baraff L. Defining normal capillary refill: variation with age, sex, and temperature. *Ann Emerg Med*. 1988;19(9):932–935.

are not always easily obtained due to a variety of factors, including noise, incorrect size of equipment, and lack of cooperation of the patient. Also note that a child may have a normal or elevated blood pressure and still be in impending shock because hypotension is a *late* finding in shock.

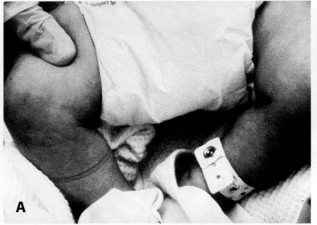
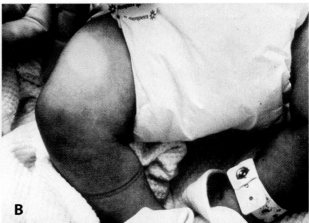

Figure 2-10 Capillary refill time is determined by compressing the skin (A) and counting the number of seconds for the skin to return to the normal color (B).

Disability

Level of consciousness, which you have already assessed in the PAT, is an excellent general assessment for neurologic status. Further assessment includes use of the AVPU scale, pupillary assessment, motor activity, and the pediatric Glasgow Coma Scale (**Tables 2-3 and 2-4**).

Table 2-3: AVPU—Neurological Assessment

ASSESSMENT	RESPONSE
A: Alert	Infant or child is alert, looking around, interactive
V: Verbal	Infant or child responds to verbal commands
P: Pain	Infant or child is responsive only to pain. May withdraw hand or moan in response to pain.
U: Unresponsive	No response to pain

Table 2-4: Pediatric Glasgow Coma Scale Scoring: Modified Scale

	CHILD	INFANT
EYES:		
4	Opens eyes spontaneously	Opens eyes spontaneously
3	Opens eyes to speech	Opens eyes to speech
2	Opens eyes to pain	Opens eyes to pain
1	NO RESPONSE	NO RESPONSE
_____ = Score (Eyes)		
MOTOR:		
6	Obeys commands	Spontaneous movements
5	Localizes	Withdraws to touch
4	Withdraws	Withdraws to pain
3	Flexion	Flexion (decorticate)
2	Extension	Extension (decerebrate)
1	NO RESPONSE	NO RESPONSE
_____ = Score (Motor)		
VERBAL:		
5	Oriented	Coos and babbles
4	Confused	Irritable cry
3	Inappropriate words	Cries to pain
2	Incomprehensible words	Moans to pain
1	NO RESPONSE	NO RESPONSE
_____ = Score (Verbal)		
_____ = Total Score (Eyes, Motor, Verbal)		
Scores will range from 3 to 15.		

Source: James HE. Neurologic evalution and support in the child with an acute brain insult. *Pediatr Ann.* Jan 1986;15(1):16–22.

AVPU

Observe whether the child is:

- *Alert*
- Responsive to *Verbal* stimuli
- Responsive only to *Pain*
- *Unresponsive*

This scoring system can be useful when assessed serially. A child may be alert as you begin your examination but may become less alert, responding only to commands (verbal stimuli). The AVPU scale gives you a very general sense of a child's neurologic status.

Glasgow Coma Scale

The Glasgow Coma Scale has been adapted for use in assessing the neurologic status of children but has *not* been validated for this use. It may be difficult to remember the scoring system, which is different for infants and children, and it may be more useful in the emergency department than in the prehospital setting.

Pupillary Assessment

Check the child's pupils with a flashlight; both pupils should constrict and be equally reactive when light is shined directly into the eyes. When the pupil is very small (pinpoint pupils), dilated, or unreactive to light, this is an abnormal finding. Abnormal pupil size may be caused by hypoxia, direct eye trauma, toxic inges-tion, damage to the brain or brainstem, or metabolic abnormalities. Note, however, that the pupils may be different sizes at baseline and that pupillary sizes are heavily dependent on ambient lighting conditions; dilated pupils in a dark environment that are briskly reactive are probably normal unless there are other indicators of neurological or toxic disease.

Motor Activity

Normal motor activity is characterized by symmetrical movement and equal strength of the extremities. Decerebrate (extension of the arms) or decorticate (flexion of the arms inward toward the chest) posturing, unusual tension or flaccidity, and seizure activity are all signs of serious neurologic problems (Figure 2-11). Always ask the caregiver about the child's normal motor function and development when making this assessment.

After assessment of the PAT and the ABCDEs you should have a good impression of how ill the child is. You should also have a general sense of the need for rapid transport and additional assistance or whether you can continue further assessment and treatment on scene. Your decision also will have to take into consideration your agency's guidelines and protocols as well as transport time to the nearest appropriate facility.

▓ Focused History and Physical Exam

When a patient is critically ill, initial assessment and critical intervention take place almost simultaneously. If the patient requires immediate transport, the focused history and physical exam can be deferred until the child is in the ambulance en route to the hospital. For small children who are not seriously ill, much of this examination can be done on the caregiver's lap. This is when you obtain a more specific picture of the possible causes of the child's illness or injury. Observe the entire body, progressing from the head to the toe of the child, including both the front and the back. For trauma patients, this examination concentrates on assessing the injuries and determining the mechanism of injury, if possible. Look for DCAP-BTLS:

- **D**eformities
- **C**ontusions
- **A**brasions
- **P**enetrating injuries
- **B**urns
- **T**enderness
- **L**acerations
- **S**welling
- Any other abnormalities

SAMPLE History

The caregiver, if available, can be of great help during the initial phase of the focused history and physical

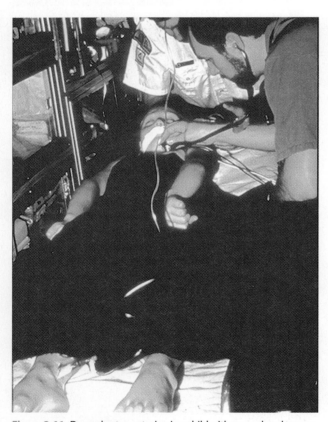

Figure 2-11 Decerebrate posturing in a child with severe head trauma.

Table 2-5: SAMPLE History

Assessment	Questions
Signs/Symptoms	What symptoms did the patient have? When did the symptoms begin? How did the patient look/feel? (See OPQRST in Table 2-6)
Allergies	Does the patient have any allergies?
Medications	Does the patient take any medications? If so, what are their names, how often taken? When was the last dose? Are any over-the-counter medications or alternative medications being taken?
Past medical history	What was the history of the birth of the child? Normal pregnancy/normal birth? Has the patient had any previous illness or hospitalizations? Has the patient had age-appropriate immunizations?
Last meal or food	When was the patient's last meal or food, including bottle- or breast-feeding?
Events leading to illness or injury	How did the illness begin? How long has the patient been ill? What caused the injury? When did the injury occur?

Table 2-6: OPQRST Assessment for Pain or Other Symptoms

Assessment	Questions
Onset	When did the pain or symptoms begin? Has the patient ever had the pain or symptoms before?
Provoke/**P**alliate	Is there anything that seems to make the pain or symptoms better or worse?
Quality	Describe the pain: Is it sharp, crampy, burning, or dull? Does it throb, or is it steady?
Region/**R**adiation	Where is the pain located? Does it seem to spread to anywhere else?
Severity	How strong is the pain or how severe are the symptoms? How has it affected your normal activities?
Time	When did the pain or symptoms begin? Are the symptoms persistent, or do they come and go?

exam by providing information about the mechanism of injury (how the injury occurred) and what happened to the child. For medical patients, try to determine the circumstances surrounding the illness, when it began, and what signs and symptoms were observed. Use the SAMPLE mnemonic to aid in performing the focused history and physical exam (Table 2-5).

For medical illness, use the mnemonic OPQRST (Table 2-6) to assess complaints and signs or symptoms.

Vital Signs

Heart Rate
Heart rates of children vary by age (Table 2-7). Count the beats for at least thirty seconds, as children's heart rates may go faster or slower along with their breathing. Assess the infant's heart rate by palpating the brachial pulse; children's pulses can be assessed at the wrist, as for an adult. The quality of the pulse also gives you important information about circulatory status of the child. Some key points:

- If the peripheral pulse is strong and regular, the child probably has adequate perfusion.
- If you cannot obtain a brachial pulse, try finding the femoral pulse and carotid pulse (in that order).
- Difficulty in palpating a carotid pulse suggests hypotension and shock.
- If no pulse can be palpated, the patient is in cardio-pulmonary arrest, unless the patient is hypothermic.

Table 2-7: Pediatric Heart Rates	
Age	Heart Rate (beats/min)
Infant	100–160
Toddler	90–150
Preschooler	80–140
School-age child	70–120
Adolescent	60–100

Respiratory Rate

Assess the infant's respiratory rate by watching the abdomen rise and fall. Infants are abdominal breathers, and it may be easier to observe the abdomen than the chest. Count the number of breaths the child takes in half a minute (thirty seconds). Because children's respiratory rates vary so much for many different reasons, counting for at least 30 seconds is likely to provide a more accurate count. Also, infants may normally stop breathing periodically ("periodic breathing") for up to 20 seconds, so a longer assessment period may be necessary to avoid an inaccurate assessment of the respiratory rate. A rate greater than 60 breaths/minute is a danger sign. When in doubt, provide supportive care.

Look for signs of respiratory distress or failure, indicated by:

- Retractions with a high respiratory rate (greater than 60 breaths/minute). The child is breathing more rapidly and with greater work of breathing in order to ensure adequate oxygenation.
- A very slow respiratory rate (less than 20 breaths/minute for a child under 6 years of age, or under 12 breaths per minute for a child 7 to 15 years of age), which can indicate respiratory failure.

Normal respiratory rates for children by age are shown in Table 2-8.

Blood Pressure

When obtaining the blood pressure, use the correct size blood pressure cuff. The width of the cuff should be equal to two thirds of the distance between the shoulder and the elbow. Children are able to compensate for

Table 2-8: Pediatric Respiratory Rates	
Age	Normal Respiratory Rate
Infant	30–60
Toddler	24–40
Preschooler	22–34
School-Age child	18–30
Adolescent	12–16

Adapted from: Dieckmann RA, Brownstein D, Gausche-Hill M (eds). *Pediatric Education for Prehospital Professionals.* Jones and Bartlett Publishers: Sudbury, MA: 2000;39.

blood loss by constriction of blood vessels and increased heart rate, and may thus be able to maintain normal blood pressure for a considerable length of time. This period is called "compensated shock."

If you can easily obtain the child's blood pressure, serial blood pressure monitoring can be helpful in determining if the child's condition is improving or deteriorating. Serial blood pressures are more useful than just one measurement. Blood pressure assessment should always be placed in the context of other measurements of circulatory status including:

- Heart rate
- Quality of pulse
- Skin temperature
- Capillary refill time

Weight

The best means of estimating the weight of a child is by using a color-coded, length-based resuscitation tape (Figure 2-12). Weight is an important assessment because the dosages of medications are determined by the weight of the child. With children who have had recent physicals or medical care, the child's caregiver may have an accurate weight.

Another method for determining weight is through use of a formula such as multiplying the age (in years) by 2 and adding 8 to 10 = Weight in kg.

If you combine the findings from the focused history and physical exam with your earlier assessments, you will have a good overall picture of the child's condition.

Where's the Evidence?

Length-based Resuscitation Tape

The use of the length-based resuscitation tape has been found to be more accurate in estimating weight than weight estimates made by experienced pediatric health care providers (physician and nurses). In a study of 937 children, Lubitz et al found that the Broselow Tape estimated weight within a 10% error rate in 85% of children, whereas only 47% of the estimates by pediatric nurses and residents were within this error range. They also found that the length-based tape was less accurate in predicting true weight of children over 25 kg.

1. Lubitz DS, Seidel JS, Chameides L, et al. A rapid method for estimating weight and resuscitation drug dosages from length in the pediatric age group. *Ann Emerg Med.* 1988;17:6:576–581.

Procedure Step-by-Step

video The steps for using a length-based resuscitation tape are described below and in Skill Drill 2-1.

1. Place the patient in the supine position and unfold the tape.
2. Place the tape next to the patient, ensuring that side A (multicolored side) is facing up.
3. Place the red end of the tape (arrow) even with the top of the patient's head, holding it there with one hand.
4. Starting from the head, run the edge of your free hand down the tape, stopping with the heel of the foot. Note the letter or color block (on edge of tape) and the weight range where your free hand has stopped, corresponding to the weight range of the child.
5. Determine the patient's weight, appropriate equipment sizes, and drug dosages from the tape and communicate this information to your colleague.

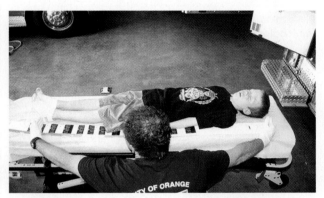

Figure 2-12 Measurement of a child using the length-based resuscitation tape to estimate weight.

Detailed Physical Exam

The detailed physical exam gives you an opportunity to take a closer look at all anatomic areas, with specific attention to any problem areas noted in your initial physical exam. You should perform this exam after the completion of critical interventions, usually en route to the receiving facility. Here are the steps for the detailed physical exam:

- Remove or lift the child's clothing to expose each area, while being careful to maintain modesty and minimize exposure to cold temperatures.
- Inspect and gently palpate any deformities, swelling, and tender or sensitive areas.
- Allow the caregiver to assist in this process by comforting and reassuring the child.

Some guidelines for observations are included in Table 2-9.

Table 2-9: Detailed Physical Exam (Head-to-Toe Assessment)	
Area	Observations
Head	Look for signs of trauma such as bruising, swelling, abrasions. Observe fontanelles in infants (closed? open? bulging? depressed?).
Mouth	Note smell of the breath. Observe for loose teeth. Note color of mucous membranes.
Neck	Observe position of trachea—midline? Listen for sounds of breathing to determine origin of upper airway sounds.
Chest	Inspect for injuries (bruises, abrasions, etc.). Palpate for deformities, broken ribs, tenderness. Observe for retractions. Repeat lung sounds.
Back	Look for signs of trauma (as above). Observe skin color. Inspect for rashes, discoloration.
Abdomen	Observe whether there is distention. Palpate gently for tenderness or masses. Auscultate for bowel sounds.
Extremities	Observe movement of extremities for symmetry. Look at color, feel temperature. Check quality pulses and sensation.

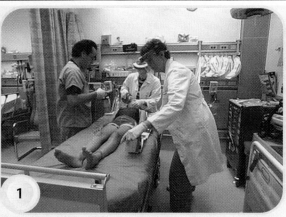

1 Place the patient in the supine position and unfold the tape.

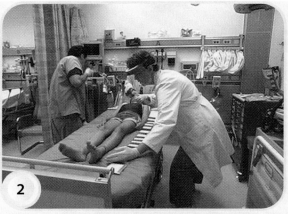

2 Place the tape next to the patient, ensuring that side A (multicolored side) is facing up.

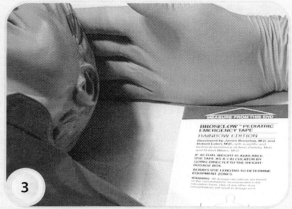

3 Place the red end of the tape (arrow) even with the top of the patient's head, holding it there with one hand.

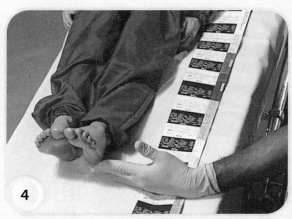

4 Starting from the head, run the edge of your free hand down the tape, stopping with the heel of the foot. Note the letter or color block (on edge of tape) and the weight range where your free hand has stopped, corresponding to the weight range of the child.

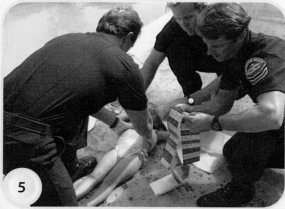

5 Determine the patient's weight, appropriate equipment sizes, and drug dosages from the tape and communicate these to your colleague.

Ongoing Assessment

Once you have completed the detailed physical exam, continue to observe the child for changes and responses to any treatments given. In some cases, you may find new problems or observe deterioration or improvements in the child's condition. Ongoing assessment should include review of the PAT, ABCDEs, repeat vital signs, and observation of the child's overall condition.

Conclusions

Assessment of the pediatric patient with respiratory compromise includes use of the Pediatric Assessment Triangle to obtain an initial impression and to determine if there is a need for immediate intervention. Further assessment includes the ABCDEs, followed by the Focused History and Detailed Physical Exam. Assessment and intervention often occur simultaneously when the child is critically ill or injured, and in-depth assessment may be made en route to the hospital. Early recognition of respiratory distress and failure is essential to a good outcome.

Scenario Review

You received a call to go to the park where you found a 2-year-old girl whose mother said the child was having difficulty breathing.

1. *How would you begin your assessment?*

Begin with the PAT. Her appearance is normal. She is alert and interactive. You note intercostal retractions and an increased respiratory rate. Her color is normal. On further assessment of ABCDEs she is found to have an open airway without stridor, wheezing in all lung fields, a rapid and strong pulse, and an appropriate level of interactivity. She has no signs of trauma or rash. She has a history of asthma.

2. *How do you determine the seriousness of the patient's condition?*

From assessment of this patient using the PAT you note that she has normal appearance and circulation but an increased work of breathing. These findings indicate that she is in respiratory distress. The ABCDEs reveal that she has signs of lower airway obstruction (wheezing) and confirm that the patient shows no signs of respiratory failure at this time. You begin treatment on-scene with supplemental oxygen and albuterol by metered dose inhaler (MDI) or nebulizer. You transport her to the hospital, performing the focused and detailed physical exam en route. After two further treatments with albuterol in the hospital, she is breathing much more easily and is discharged home.

Quick Quiz

1. *The Pediatric Assessment Triangle consists of:*

A. Breathing, Circulation, and Level of Consciousness

B. Airway, Breathing, and Circulation

C. Appearance, Work of Breathing, and Level of Consciousness

D. Airway, Breathing, and Level of Consciousness

E. Appearance, Work of Breathing, and Circulatory Status

2. *A two year-old patient is probably not seriously ill if he/she:*

A. Is alert and responds interactively

B. Has a normal blood pressure and heart rate

C. Has a respiratory rate greater than 15 breaths/min

D. Has skin mottling with a normal respiratory rate

E. Is awake and has a normal blood pressure

3. *Which of the following is a true statement?*

A. Respiratory rates of children are similar to those of adults.

B. Respiratory rates of children can be affected by diet, temperature, and lack of sleep.

C. Respiratory rates of children should be counted for 15 seconds for an accurate assessment.

D. Children are not able to increase their respiratory rates in response to hypoxia.

E. A higher than normal respiratory rate with increased work of breathing is a danger sign.

4. *Your general impression of a child in respiratory distress would be based on the assessment of which of the following signs or symptoms?*

A. Skin redness

B. Dilated pupils

C. Moist skin

D. Retractions

E. Extremity pain

5. *Which of the following signs suggests an upper airway obstruction?*

A. Wheezing

B. Rales

C. Crackles

D. Stridor

E. Rhonchi

Glossary

accessory muscles   Muscles that assist in respiration.

acrocyanosis   Cyanosis of the extremities; this may be normal in the hands and feet of an infant within the first hour after birth.

alveoli   The air sacs of the lungs in which the exchange of oxygen and carbon dioxide takes place.

bronchi   The two main branches leading from the trachea to the lungs, providing the passageway for air movement.

bronchioles   The smaller air passages in the lungs that extend from the bronchi to the alveoli.

crackles   A series of short nonmusical sounds heard during inspiration, also called rales.

cyanosis   Slightly bluish, grayish, slatelike, or dark purple discoloration of the skin due to the presence of hypoxia.

hypoxia Inadequate oxygen.

intercostal Between the ribs.

Pediatric Assessment Triangle An assessment tool for obtaining an immediate general impression of the seriousness of an illness or injury by focusing on visual and auditory clues about general appearance, work of breathing, and circulatory status of the infant or child.

rales A series of short nonmusical sounds heard during inspiration; also called crackles.

retractions Physical drawing in of the chest wall that occurs with increased work of breathing.

rhonchi A dry, low-pitched sound caused by partial obstruction of the airway.

substernal Situated beneath the sternum.

supraclavicular Located above the clavicle.

Selected References

1. Dieckmann RA, Brownstein D, Gausche-Hill M (eds). *Pediatric Education for Prehospital Professionals: PEPP Textbook,* Jones & Bartlett Publishers, Sudbury, MA, 2000;39, 58–77.

2. Gausche M, Henderson DP, Seidel JS. Vital signs as a part of the prehospital assessment of the pediatric patient: A survey of paramedics. *Ann Emerg Med.* 1990; 19:173–178.

3. Gausche-Hill M, Dieckmann RA, Brownstein D (eds). *Pediatric Education for Prehospital Professionals: PEPP Resource Manual,* Jones & Bartlett Publishers, Sudbury, MA, 2000;60–71.

4. Gorelick MH, Shaw KN, Baker MD. Effect of ambient temperature on capillary refill in healthy children. *Pediatrics.* 1993;92(5):699–702.

5. James HE. Neurologic evalution and support in the child with an acute brain insult. *Pediatr Ann.* Jan 1986;15(1):16–22.

6. Lubitz DS, Seidel JSS, Chameides L, et al. A rapid method for estimating weight and resuscitation drug dosages from length in the pediatric age group. *Ann Emerg Med.* 1988;17:6:576–581.

7. Schriger DL, Baraff L. Defining normal capillary refill: variation with age, sex, and temperature. *Ann Emerg Med.* 1988;19(9):932–935.

End of Chapter Activities

Technology Resources

Online Course

Anatomy Review

Online Glossary

Web Links

Online Quiz

Scenarios

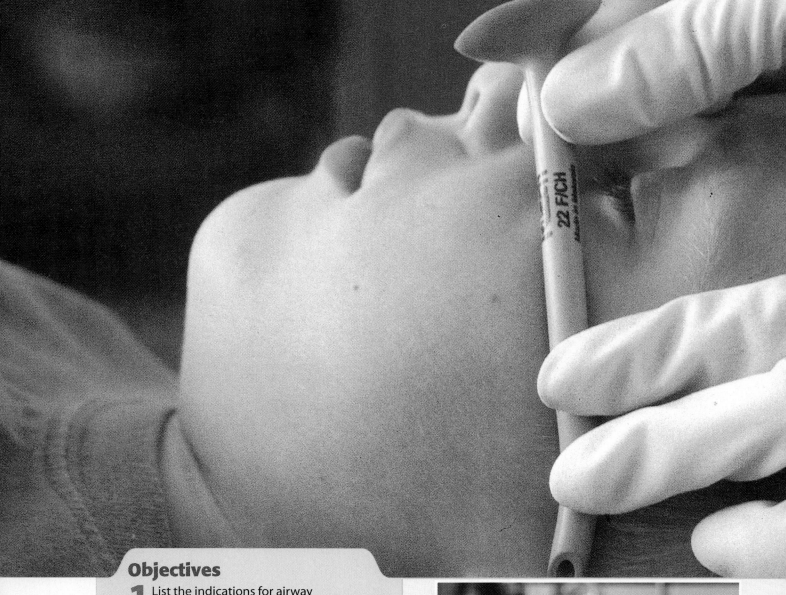

Objectives

1 List the indications for airway management of the pediatric patient.

2 Prioritize airway management procedures based on the assessment.

3 Identify purposes for and types of monitoring devices available for use in the prehospital setting.

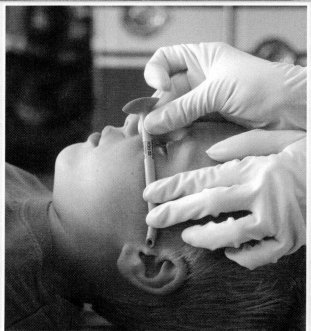

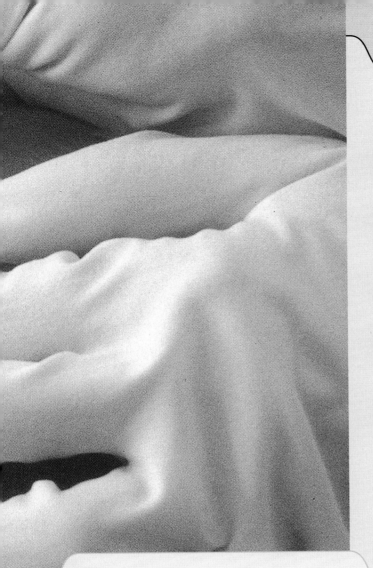

CHAPTER 3

Managing the Pediatric Airway in a Step-by-Step Approach

Scenario

You are called to the home of a 6-month-old male with difficulty breathing. When you arrive the infant is lethargic, with pale skin, decreased respiratory rate, and poor tidal volume. Your general impression is that the infant is in respiratory failure.

1. *What are your management priorities for this patient?*

2. *How would you support ventilation and oxygenation for this patient?*

Think about these questions and this case as you read on. We will return to this scenario at the end of the chapter.

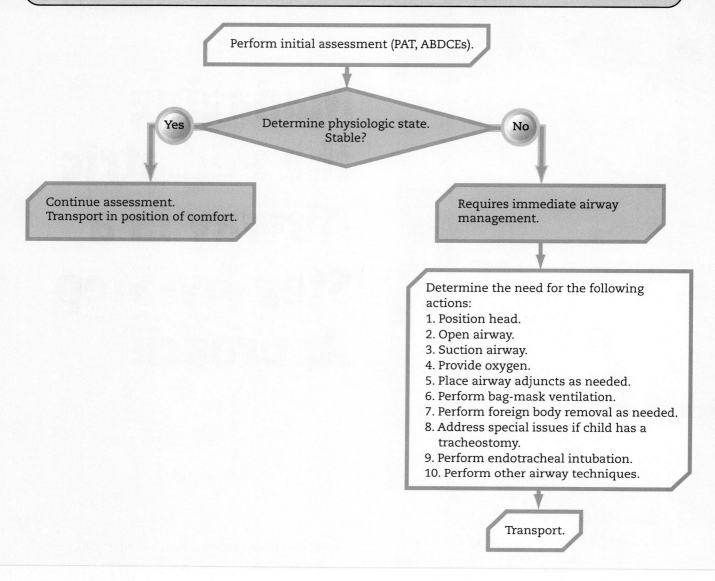

Perform initial assessment (PAT, ABDCEs).

Determine physiologic state. Stable?

Yes → Continue assessment. Transport in position of comfort.

No → Requires immediate airway management.

Determine the need for the following actions:
1. Position head.
2. Open airway.
3. Suction airway.
4. Provide oxygen.
5. Place airway adjuncts as needed.
6. Perform bag-mask ventilation.
7. Perform foreign body removal as needed.
8. Address special issues if child has a tracheostomy.
9. Perform endotracheal intubation.
10. Perform other airway techniques.

Transport.

■ Introduction

Airway management should proceed in a stepwise fashion based on the assessment of the infant or child. Assessment includes taking an appropriate history and evaluating the patient for physical signs and symptoms that give clues to the underlying cause of respiratory distress or failure. Management priorities will be driven by this assessment. For example, the management priorities are very different for a child with <u>wheezing</u> versus <u>stridor</u> or for a child with signs of respiratory distress versus respiratory failure.

The first step in airway management is assessment of <u>physiologic status</u> and possible etiology (cause). If the patient is determined to be in respiratory failure then immediate management is needed to support oxygenation and ventilation. This man-

agement proceeds in a stepwise fashion from simple head positioning maneuvers to advanced airway management.

Airway management in the prehospital setting has been traditionally viewed and taught as a series of individual skills. How these skills relate to one another to form an airway management plan for the patient has not been emphasized. To support the concept of an airway management plan for patients, consider:

- The recognized indications for airway management techniques.
- The success rate and complication rate of those techniques.
- The effect on patient outcome associated with each skill.

Where's the Evidence?

Efficacy of BLS Airway Maneuvers

In a study of airway management in children in Los Angeles and Orange Counties, California, a combination of basic airway maneuvers including positioning the head, opening the airway, suctioning, placing oropharyngeal and nasopharyngeal airways, followed by bag-mask ventilation was as effective as endotracheal intubation in creating positive outcomes for children with respiratory or cardiopulmonary failure. In fact, in children with respiratory failure alone, basic airway management alone led to improved survival. Advanced life support maneuvers to remove a foreign body obstructing the airway were also life-saving in this study. However, children who received bag-mask ventilation after the foreign object was removed had better neurologic function than those who received endotracheal intubation. From these data we know that basic airway management is often all that is necessary to support oxygenation and ventilation in the pediatric patient.

The recent revision of the EMT-Basic and paramedic National Standard curriculum supports a graded approach to airway management, as does the Pediatric Education for Prehospital Professionals (PEPP) Course and the previous edition of the *Pediatric Airway Management Course*.

1. Dieckmann RA, Brownstein D, Gausche-Hill M (eds). *Pediatric Education for Prehospital Professionals: PEPP Textbook,* Jones & Bartlett Publishers, Sudbury, MA, 2000.
2. Gausche-Hill M, Dieckmann RA, Brownstein D (eds). *Pediatric Education for Prehospital Professionals: PEPP Resource Manual,* Jones & Bartlett Publishers, Sudbury, MA, 2000.
3. Gausche M, Lewis RJ, Stratton SJ. Effect of out-of-hospital pediatric endotracheal intubation on survival and neurological outcome: A controlled clinical trial. *JAMA.* 2000;283:6:783–790.
4. *Student Manual: Pediatric Airway Management Project;* 1st and 2nd edition, funded by Maternal and Child Health Bureau in Collaboration with the National Highway Traffic and Safety Administration, 1993, 1995.
5. Gausche M, Goodrich SM, Poore PD: *Instructor Manual for Advanced Life Support Providers: Pediatric Airway Management Project;* 1st and 2nd edition, includes full slide set, funded by Maternal and Child Health Bureau in collaboration with the National Highway Traffic and Safety Administration and the Agency for Healthcare Research and Quality, first edition, 1993; second edition, 1997.
6. *Emergency Medical Technician Paramedic: National Standard Curriculum* (EMT-P), 1998, National Highway Traffic Safety Administration. (http://www.nhtsa.dot.gov/people/injury/ems/EMT-P/)

Anatomical Considerations

video All airway anatomical, physiological, and behavioral differences between adults and children noted in the discussion in Chapter 1 affect airway management strategies. These differences are important in initial assessment, equipment selection, and skills to be used in management.

Indications

Indications for pediatric airway management include the following:
- Respiratory distress
- Respiratory failure
- Respiratory arrest
- Decompensated shock (shock associated with low blood pressure as compensatory mechanisms fail)
- Cardiopulmonary failure
- Cardiopulmonary arrest
- Neurologic resuscitation for patients with signs of severe head trauma
- Airway at risk for subsequent obstruction, as in airway burns (airway edema leading to obstruction) or severe overdose (protection of the airway when airway reflexes are blunted)

Airway management includes a wide spectrum of activities. Indications for airway management as listed above may require basic maneuvers such as head positioning, suctioning, and opening the airway, or more complex interventions such as bag-mask ventilation, endotracheal intubation, or cricothyrotomy. Begin management using basic skills with a low risk of complications, and if needed, proceed to higher-risk procedures. Initial interventions will always include positioning the head, opening the airway, and providing supplemental oxygen. When this level of intervention is completed, reassess the need for further intervention. If needed, continue management by performing suctioning, placing airway adjuncts, providing bag-mask ventilation, or using BLS foreign body removal procedures. At this point, reassess the patient to determine the need for more advanced airway procedures including endotracheal intubation, ALS foreign body removal procedures, or cricothyrotomy.

Contraindications

Contraindications for airway management include the assessment that the patient has adequate oxygenation and ventilation and is not at risk for deterioration.

- Adequate oxygenation and ventilation
- No need to protect the airway
- No evidence of severe head trauma

Procedure Step-by-Step

video Airway management should proceed based on assessment (Chapter 2: Assessment). Each airway management step is followed by a reassessment of the patient to ensure that the intervention has improved the patient's clinical status.

The following is a list of graduated airway management skills. Not every skill will be needed on every patient:

1. Perform the initial assessment including the Pediatric Assessment Triangle and ABCDEs.

2. Determine the physiologic state: stable or requires immediate airway management (respiratory distress, respiratory failure, respiratory arrest, cardiopulmonary failure, cardiopulmonary arrest).

3. Determine the need for the following actions based on level of respiratory dysfunction:

   a. Position the head in the midline position with a towel under the shoulders or head, as appropriate, to level the plane of the airway. Open the airway by performing a head tilt-chin lift in a medical patient or jaw-thrust maneuver in a trauma patient (Figures 3-1 and 3-2).

   b. Suction the airway (Figure 3-3).

   c. Provide oxygen supplementation, either by blow-by or partial nonrebreather mask or by bag-mask ventilation (Figure 3-4).

   d. Place airway adjuncts, such as a nasopharyngeal airway (semiconscious patient) or an oropharyngeal airway (unconscious patient without a gag reflex) (Figure 3-5).

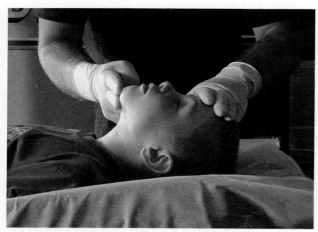

Figure 3-1 Head tilt-chin lift maneuver to open the airway.

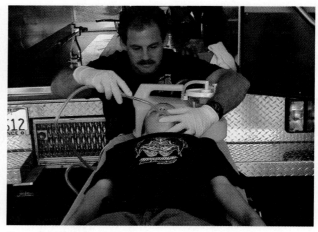

Figure 3-3 Suction the airway.

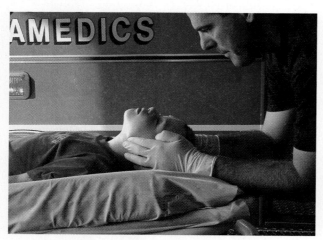

Figure 3-2 Jaw-thrust maneuver to open the airway.

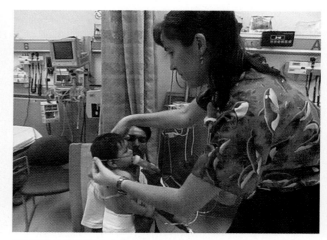

Figure 3-4 Provide supplemental oxygen.

e. Perform bag-mask ventilation to provide support of ventilation and oxygenation for patients requiring assisted ventilation or neurological resuscitation (Figure 3-6).

f. Perform endotracheal intubation if this skill is within the scope of practice in your EMS system, and if bag-mask ventilation is unsuccessful in improving the patient's clinical status (Figure 3-7).

g. Perform other airway techniques, depending on the assessment of the patient (i.e., laryngoscopy and use of pediatric Magill forceps to remove foreign body, laryngeal mask airway, or needle cricothyrotomy) (Figure 3-8).

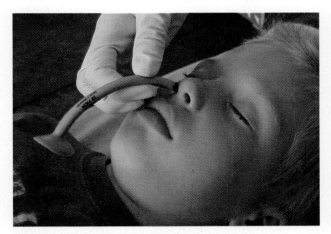

Figure 3-5 Placing a nasopharyngeal airway.

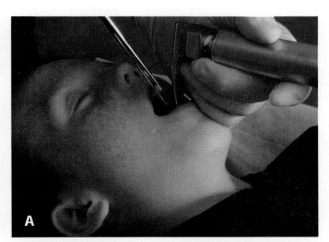

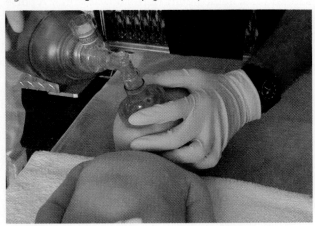

Figure 3-6 Bag-mask ventilation.

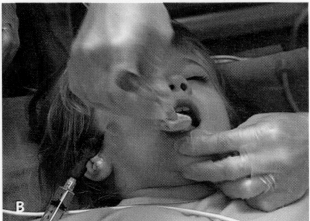

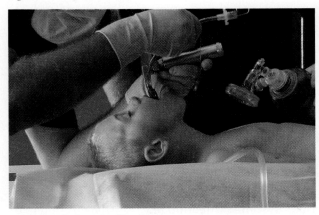

Figure 3-7 Endotracheal intubation.

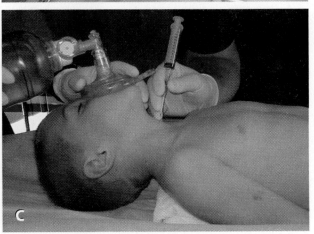

Figure 3-8 (A) Laryngoscopy and use of Magill forceps to remove a quarter; (B) Laryngeal mask airway; (C) Needle cricothyrotomy.

Your airway management plan should be based on the degree and type of respiratory dysfunction of the patient. For example, for a patient with seizures and gurgling airway sounds, your assessment suggests a partial upper airway obstruction. Positioning the head in the midline, suctioning the airway, and placing a nasopharyngeal airway would be appropriate steps in your initial airway management plan for this patient. If after reassessment, the abnormal airway sounds resolve and the patient's color improves, there would be no need to move to additional steps.

In another case, the Pediatric Assessment Triangle may reveal a child with a history of asthma who is unconscious, apneic, and pale. You conclude that the child is in respiratory failure. Positioning the head, opening the airway, and performing bag-mask ventilation with 100% oxygen would be the appropriate initial steps in your airway management.

As illustrated above, the order of the steps in the airway management plan may vary with your assessment of the clinical status of the patient. The application of the plan for these assessments is shown in Figures 3-9 and 3-10, as well as in the Pediatric Airway Management Algorithm presented at the beginning of this chapter.

TRICKS
of the Trade

1. Begin with assessment of the adequacy of ventilation and oxygenation. This assessment will drive your airway management plan.

2. Airway management should proceed in an orderly process beginning with positioning the head. Each step in airway management is dependent on appropriate performance of the previous step. If the skills are not performed sequentially, each subsequent procedure will be less effective.

3. Reassess the patient after each intervention to ensure that your intervention has resulted in improvement in the patient's clinical status.

4. Remember the airway management algorithm as shown at the beginning of this chapter. This will help to organize your thoughts, reduce anxiety in performing skills, and give you greater self-efficacy for skill performance.

Complications

Complications of interventions include the following:
- Hypoxia/anoxia (inadequate or complete lack of oxygenation)
- Vomiting
- Aspiration
- Upper airway trauma including bleeding into the airway or tooth lodged in the airway

- Vocal cord trauma or damage to trachea below the vocal cords
- Spinal injury

Every skill has a risk of complications as described in subsequent chapters. It is important to weigh the risks versus the benefits of the procedures. The most appropriate airway management skill is one that provides treatment for the physiologic derangement and is associated with the lowest risk of complications.

Monitoring

During transport, continue to assess the patient with pulse oximetry, electrocardiographic (ECG) monitoring, and exhaled carbon dioxide (CO_2) monitoring as available. Remember to integrate your clinical assessment with the results of objective monitoring devices.

Pulse oximetry uses infrared technology to measure the oxygen saturation in the blood. These devices have sensors that look like adhesive bandages or small clips placed over the end of a finger or toe (Figure 3-11); oxygen saturation values are displayed on a digital monitor (Figure 3-12). Pulse oximetry is a simple noninvasive method of monitoring the degree of oxygen saturation of hemoglobin. Here's how it works: A pulse oximeter probe is attached to the patient, usually to the finger or toe, although any reasonably translucent site with good blood flow may be used. This probe uses a light emitter that shines through the site to a photodetector that receives the light. The light is partly absorbed by hemoglobin, in amounts which differ according to the saturation with oxygen. By measuring the absorption, the proportion of oxygenated hemoglobin is calculated.

When using pulse oximetry in clinical practice, ask yourself these three questions:
- Is the patient adequately oxygenating?
- Is the patient adequately ventilating?
- Could the patient's condition prevent adequate gas exchange in the lung?

Is the patient adequately oxygenating? If not, add supplemental oxygen. Normal pulse oximetry readings are between 96 and 100%. Once the oxygen saturation level drops to less than 94%, supplemental oxygen should be added. Remember also that pulse oximetry measures only the oxygenation of blood and does not provide information about ventilation. Also note that based on physiologic principles, a patient with an oxygen saturation level in the 90 to 92% range can quickly drop to the low 80% range with only a slight drop in ventilation.

Is the patient adequately ventilating? If not, begin assisted ventilation. Remember that a patient can have normal oxygenation and poor ventilation (for example, a patient with muscular weakness from a serious systemic infection (e.g., sepsis), botulism, or

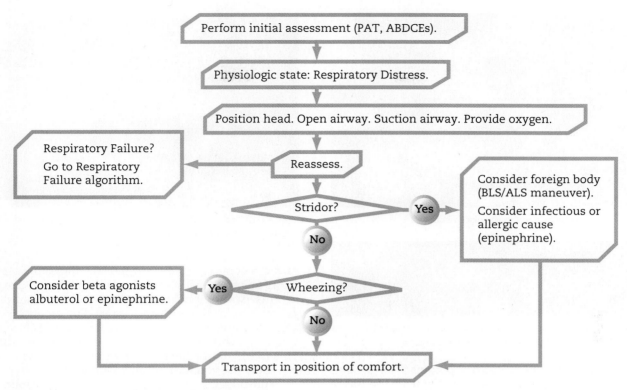

Figure 3-9 Management of respiratory distress.

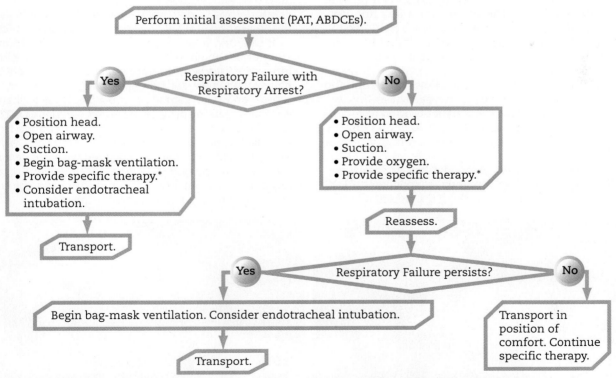

*Specific therapy depends on the cause. For a foreign body, perform BLS/ALS foreign body removal procedures; for wheezing, administer albuterol and epinephrine; for stridor, administer epinephrine.

Figure 3-10 Management of respiratory failure.

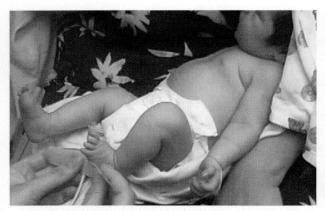

Figure 3-11 Pulse oximetry probe placement.

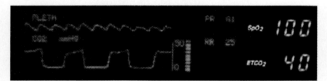

Figure 3-12 Oxygen saturation monitor showing waveform correlating with pulse and digital readout of oxygen saturation.

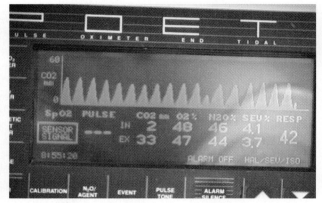

Figure 3-13 End-tidal CO_2 monitor showing digital readout of inhaled and exhaled CO_2 concentration.

muscular dystrophy. It is also important to realize that because there is an oxygen reservoir in the nasopharynx, oropharynx, and airways, pulse oximetry values can be maintained for several minutes even after breathing ceases. This oxygen reservoir can provide sufficient oxygen to the tissues for a few minutes. Oxygen saturation values alone cannot be utilized to determine when bag-mask ventilation should be initiated or continued; these decisions must be guided by clinical assessment.

Pulse oximetry also helps to identify patients who are hypoxemic or whose blood oxygen saturation levels are dangerously low. These patients often have conditions that prevent adequate gas exchange in the lung, such as pneumonia, submersion injury, or pulmonary edema.

What other monitoring modalities can assist you in determining the need for airway management? ECG monitoring can be used to assess if the patient is brady-cardic, a common finding in the late stages of respiratory failure. Respiratory failure with bradycardia represents cardiopulmonary failure and may rapidly progress to cardiopulmonary arrest. The prognosis of a patient in respiratory failure is far better (80% survival) than with cardiopulmonary arrest (9% survival). This is why immediate intervention to support oxygenation and ventilation can be life-saving.

End-tidal CO_2 detectors or capnographs (capnography refers to the specific devices that produce a waveform) are used to confirm the placement of an endotracheal tube in the trachea (Figure 3-13). The colorimetric CO_2 detector devices are commonly used in the prehospital setting. This type of CO_2 detector as illustrated in Figure 3-14 is attached to the 15 mm adapter of the endotracheal tube after endotracheal intubation has been completed. When the patient inhales or when oxygen flows past the paper sensor, the sensor retains its original color (purple). If gas exchange is occurring in the lungs, the patient exhales CO_2. This is detected by the sensor causing color change from the baseline purple color to a yellow or tan color. A yellow or tan color change is associated with tracheal intubation and purple indicates possible esophageal intubation. CO_2 detection and monitoring will be covered in Chapter 7: Endotracheal Intubation.

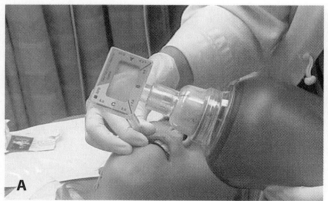
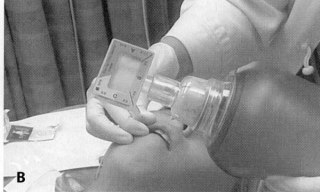

Figure 3-14 The end-tidal CO_2 detector is placed on the end of the tracheal tube to measure presence of exhaled CO_2. (A) shows purple with oxygen flowing through the sensor with ventilation and (B) shows the device detecting CO_2 (yellow) with exhalation.

Conclusions

Airway management is a process involving clinical assessment followed by graduated interventions and re-assessment. Basic airway management serves as the foundation. Advanced airway management is added to this foundation after careful assessment of the patient's condition and determination that the benefit of more advanced procedures outweighs the potential risk. More research is needed to help determine the effect of these procedures on patient outcome.

Scenario Review

You were called to the home of a 6-month-old male with difficulty breathing. Your general impression was that the infant was in respiratory failure.

1. *What are your initial treatment priorities?*

Place the infant in the supine position and open the airway using either jaw-thrust or head tilt-chin lift maneuver. Begin bag-mask ventilation with 100% oxygen and then reassess adequacy of ventilation. There is adequate chest rise with bag-mask ventilation and pulse oximetry reads 94%. The ECG monitor initially showed a pulse rate of 70 beats per minute, which has increased with your ventilation to 120 beats per minute. The infant's color has improved.

Airway management for this patient can be summarized by the following steps:

- Position the head, keep head midline, and place a small towel under the shoulders.
- Open the airway.
- Determine the appropriate-sized equipment.
- Measure mask and begin bag-mask ventilation.
- Begin monitoring (ECG, pulse oximetry).
- Reassess – look for chest rise and fall and improvement in patient's condition.
- If no chest rise, reposition, suction, consider airway adjunct.
- Consider further airway management as needed.

2. *How would you support ventilation and oxygenation for this patient?*

- Position the head. Airway obstruction from a flexed head on the neck or head tilt to the side positioning is averted through good positioning.
- Provide 100% oxygen by bag-mask ventilation technique.

You continue bag-mask ventilation and consider the option of endotracheal intubation for this patient. Transport time to the nearest pediatric receiving facility is 10 minutes. Because the infant's condition has improved with basic airway management and supplemental oxygen, you determine that the risk of complications associated with further intervention including endotracheal intubation is greater than the potential benefit it may provide given the short transport time. After arrival in the emergency department, the patient's condition continues to improve and bag-mask ventilation is discontinued. It is determined that the infant suffered a febrile seizure and respiratory failure from lack of muscle tone. Your intervention was both appropriate and life-saving for this patient.

Quick Quiz

1. *You are called to the home of a 20-month-old female with a seizure. The toddler has a history of fever for one day and the mother noted the toddler was unresponsive with twitching of her hands and feet. You arrive and note the following: the toddler is unconscious and seizing with foam coming from her mouth; she has good rise and fall of the chest without retractions; her color is pale; and there is a bluish hue around her mouth. What are your first three initial management steps?*

   A. Position the head, suction, add supplemental oxygen.
   B. Suction, place an IV, perform endotracheal intubation.
   C. Place a nasopharyngeal airway, begin bag-mask ventilation, place on a monitor.
   D. Place an oropharyngeal airway, suction, add supplemental oxygen.

2. *You are called to the home of a 3-month-old female found lifeless in the crib by her mother. When you arrive, the parents are frantically trying to perform CPR. You gently ask them to step aside so you can assess their child and note that the infant is unconscious, there are no spontaneous respirations, and her color is pale. You feel for a pulse and none is present. What are the first three steps in the management of this infant?*

   A. Position the head, open the airway, begin bag-mask ventilation.
   B. Suction, place an oropharyngeal airway, provide supplemental oxygen by face mask.
   C. Position the head, suction, perform endotracheal intubation.
   D. Open the airway, use laryngoscopy and Magill forceps to assess for possible foreign body aspiration.

3. *A 4-year-old male ate a hard candy at a company picnic. Bystanders note he grabbed his throat and fell to the ground. Your response time is 1 minute. On your arrival the bystanders are trying to remove the candy and are performing rescue ventilation. Your assessment shows the boy is not breathing but has a strong*

pulse. What are the first three steps in your management of this patient?

    A. Suction, place an oropharyngeal airway, add supplemental oxygen by mask.

    B. Suction, attempt bag-mask ventilation, and then perform endotracheal intubation around the obstruction.

    C. Position the head, perform bag-mask ventilation, if no chest rise, perform immediate cricothyrotomy.

    D. Open the airway and look to see if the candy is visible, and if so, remove it; if not attempt bag-mask ventilation; if no chest rise, then perform 5 abdominal thrusts.

4. *Choose the best statement describing the process of pediatric airway management.*

    A. Perform the most advanced airway maneuver first to save time.

    B. Perform assessment followed by a graduated series of skills and reassessment.

    C. Perform only those skills that you feel confident in performing.

    D. Perform only skills with the lowest risk.

Glossary

airway adjunct　An artificial device to maintain an open airway.

aspiration　The process of sucking in. Foreign bodies may be aspirated into the nose, throat, or lungs on inspiration.

botulism　Food poisoning from consuming the bacterium *Clostridium botulinum* from spoiled food; illness is characterized by motor problems, visual problems, and dryness (for example, of airway).

capnograph　A device used to confirm placement of an endotracheal tube; displays exhaled CO_2 in graph form.

cardiopulmonary arrest　A state in which no respiration and circulation are occuring; the patient is apneic and pulseless on examination.

cardiopulmonary failure　A state of inadequate respiration and circulation during which there is no breathing and no pulse.

colorimetric CO_2 detector　An instrument that determines the amount of carbon dioxide in expired air; measurements are represented by colors.

decompensated shock　Shock associated with low blood pressure as compensatory mechanisms fail.

head tilt-chin lift　A maneuver used to open the airway of a medical patient; in this maneuver, the forehead is tilted back and the chin is simultaneously lifted.

hypoxemic　Characterized by having deficient oxygenation in the blood.

jaw-thrust maneuver　A maneuver that can be used to open the airway of a trauma or medical patient; in this maneuver, two fingers are placed behind the angle of the jaw and the jaw is brought forward.

muscular dystrophy　An inherited condition involving weakness and atrophy of the muscles.

partial nonrebreather mask　A mask that adds a reservoir bag to increase inspired oxygen to 60%.

physiologic status　State of a person's body functioning.

pulse oximetry　The measurement of oxygen saturation in the blood through the use of infrared technology; the device is clipped over the end of a finger or toe and oxygen saturation levels are displayed on a digital monitor.

stridor　A harsh sound during inspiration, high-pitched due to partial upper airway obstruction.

wheezing　Production of whistling sounds during expiration such as occurs in asthma and bronchiolitis.

Selected References

1. American Heart Association. guidelines for cardiopulmonary resuscitation and emergency cardiovascular care: Pediatric basic life support and pediatric advanced life support. *Circulation.* 2000;102(8):I-253–I-342.

2. Bass JL, Mehta KA. Oxygen desaturation of selected term infants in car seats. *Pediatrics.* 1995;96:288–290.

3. Bhende MS, Thompson AE. Evaluation of an end-tidal CO_2 detector during pediatric cardiopulmonary resuscitation. *Pediatrics.* 1995;95:395–399.

4. Bhende MS, Thompson AE, Cook DR. Validity of a disposable end-tidal CO_2 detector in verifying endotracheal tube placement in infants and children. *Ann Emerg Med.* 1992;21:142–145.

5. Bhende MS, Thompson AE, Orr RA. Utility of an end-tidal carbon dioxide detector during stabilization and transport of critically ill children. *Pediatrics.* 1992;89:1042–1044.

6. Cote CJ, Rolf N, Liu LMP. A single-blind study of combined pulse oximetry and capnography in children. *Anesthesiology.* 1991;74:980–987.

7. Curley MAQ, Thompson JE. End-tidal CO_2 monitoring in critically ill infants and children. *Pediatr Nurs.* 1990;16:397–403.

8. Dieckmann RA, Brownstein D, Gausche-Hill M (eds). *Pediatric Education for Prehospital Professionals: PEPP Textbook,* Jones & Bartlett Publishers, Sudbury, MA, 2000;58–78.

9. *Emergency Medical Technician Paramedic: National Standard Curriculum* (EMT-P), 1998, National Highway Traffic Safety Administration. (http://www.nhtsa.dot.gov/people/injury/ems/EMT-P/)

10. Gausche-Hill M, Dieckmann RA, Brownstein D (eds). *Pediatric Education for Prehospital Professionals: PEPP Resource Manual,* Jones & Bartlett Publishers, Sudbury, MA, 2000;35–43, 60–71.

11. Gausche M, Lewis RJ, Stratton SJ. Effect of out-of-hospital pediatric endotracheal intubation on survival and neurological outcome: A controlled clinical trial. *JAMA.* 2000;283:6:783–790.

12. Gausche M, Goodrich SM, Poore PD. *Instructor Manual for Advanced Life Support Providers: Pediatric Airway Management Project;* Maternal and Child Health Bureau

in collaboration with the National Highway Traffic and Safety Administration and the Agency for Healthcare Research and Quality, 1997, Washington, D.C.;17–35.

13. Hayden SR, Sciammarella J, Viccellio P, Thode H, Delagi R. Colorimetric end-tidal CO_2 detector for verification of endotracheal tube placement in out-of-hospital cardiac arrest. *Acad Emerg Med.* 1995;2:499–502.

14. Lee BS, Gausche-Hill M. Pediatric airway management. *Clin Pediatr Emerg Med.* 2001; 2:2:91–106.

15. Knapp S, Kofler J, Stoiser B. The assessment of four different methods to verify tracheal tube placement in the critical care setting. *Anesth Analg.* 1999;88:766–770.

16. Short L, Hecker RB, Middaugh RE, Menk EJ. A comparison of pulse oximeters during helicopter flight. *J Emerg Med.* 1989:7:639–643.

17. *Student Manual: Pediatric Airway Management Project*; 1st and 2nd edition, funded by Maternal and Child Health Bureau in Collaboration with the National Highway Traffic and Safety Administration, 1993, 1995.

18. White RD, Asplin BR. Out-of-hospital quantitative monitoring of end-tidal carbon dioxide pressure during CPR. *Ann Emerg Med.* 1994;23:25–30.

Technology Resources

Online Course

Anatomy Review

Online Glossary

Web Links

Online Quiz

Scenarios

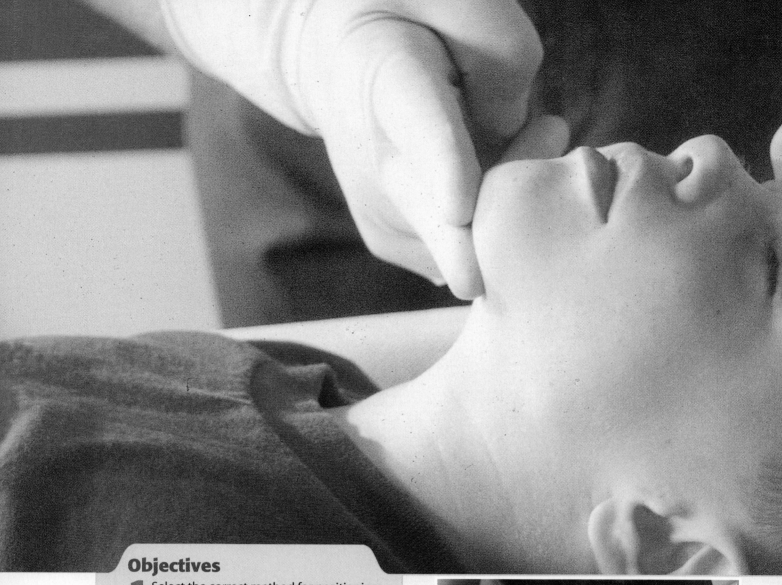

Objectives

1 Select the correct method for positioning and opening the airway of a medical and trauma patient.

2 List the indications and contraindications in the use of oropharyngeal and nasopharyngeal airways.

3 Choose the correct size oropharyngeal or nasopharyngeal airway.

4 Describe the proper sequence in placing an oropharyngeal or nasopharyngeal airway.

5 Identify complications in using oropharyngeal and nasopharyngeal airways, then determine corrective measures.

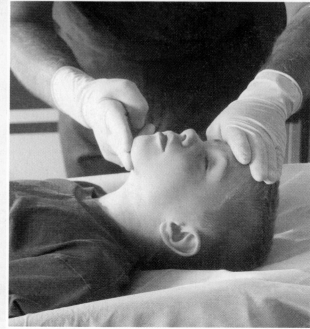

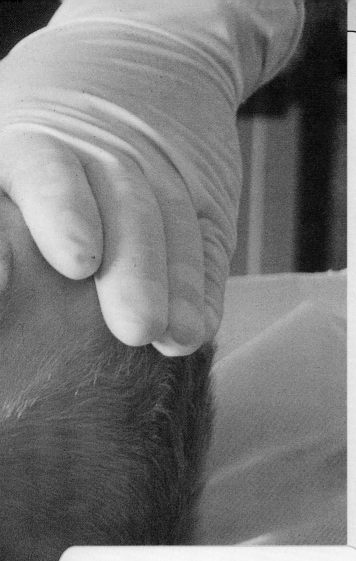

CHAPTER 4

Positioning the Patient and Opening the Airway

Scenario

You respond to an intersection where you find a 10-year-old boy who was hit by a truck as he rode his bike across the street. Upon arrival you note the boy is unresponsive with a high-pitched cry. A large forehead laceration is noted.

1. *What are your initial assessment priorities?*

2. *What are your initial treatment priorities?*

Think about these questions and this case as you read on. We will return to this scenario at the end of the chapter.

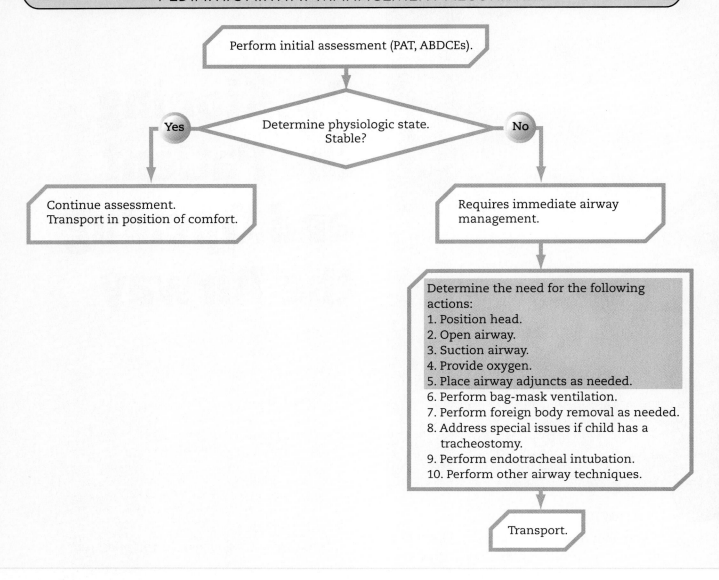

Perform initial assessment (PAT, ABDCEs).

Yes ← Determine physiologic state. Stable? → **No**

Continue assessment.
Transport in position of comfort.

Requires immediate airway management.

Determine the need for the following actions:
1. Position head.
2. Open airway.
3. Suction airway.
4. Provide oxygen.
5. Place airway adjuncts as needed.
6. Perform bag-mask ventilation.
7. Perform foreign body removal as needed.
8. Address special issues if child has a tracheostomy.
9. Perform endotracheal intubation.
10. Perform other airway techniques.

Transport.

■ Introduction

Medical and trauma patients alike can be unable to maintain a <u>patent</u> airway for a variety of reasons. Early recognition of a compromised airway can save lives and prevent disability. There are several techniques that are used to open and maintain an open airway. These include: head positioning, airway opening techniques (jaw thrust, head tilt-chin lift), and the use of airway adjuncts. Use of these simple techniques may avert the need for more invasive airway management such as bag-mask ventilation and endotracheal intubation.

The ultimate success of airway management is directly related to performing the necessary steps in proper sequence. These steps include assessment, followed by appropriate intervention, followed by reassessment.

■ Anatomical Considerations

video Anatomical considerations for positioning the patient and opening a pediatric airway include the following:

Prominent Occiput

The occiput of an infant or young child is more prominent than an adult's, thus different positioning is required to open the airway. The larger occiput of infants **(Figure 4-1A)** may cause flexion of the head on the neck. The more flexible cartilage in the trachea permits extra mobility of the trachea, which can cause bending and obstruction of the airway when the neck is flexed forward or when it is hyperextended. For correct airway positioning, the shoulders can be slightly elevated

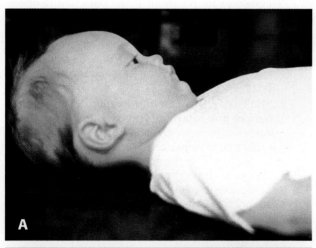
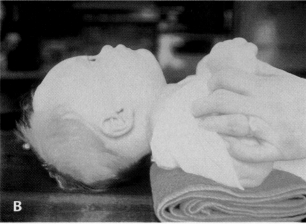

Figure 4-1 (A) Infants have a proportionally larger occiput than adults; (B) Place a small towel underneath the shoulders to achieve correct positioning.

with a small towel underneath (Figure 4-1B) and the head kept in the midline position.

Larger Tongue

The tongue of a child is larger in proportion to the size of the mouth than an adults, and, when there is loss of muscle tone, can fall back against the posterior pharynx causing upper airway obstruction. Airway adjuncts, such as nasal and oropharyngeal airways, can be used to prevent airway obstruction caused by the tongue and will allow for a clear passage of air from the environment to the posterior pharynx and the tracheal opening.

Preferential Nose Breathing

Infants are preferential nose breathers, so nasal obstruction makes breathing more difficult. Any fluid, secretions, material, or object placed in the nostril can lead to respiratory distress in young infants.

Indications

Indications for the use of airway adjuncts in pediatric patients include the following:
- Inability to maintain an open airway
  - Altered mental status
  - Loss of muscle tone
  - Airway obstruction from secretions or the tongue

Altered mental status may occur with inadequate oxygenation. As altered mental status becomes more pronounced, the patient may no longer be able to maintain a patent airway without assistance. Signs that may indicate a need for an airway adjunct include noisy or snoring respirations caused by loss of muscle tone, increased secretions, or tongue obstruction of the upper airway. With rapid and appropriate intervention, respiratory failure may be prevented. Proper positioning and use of airway adjuncts to maintain the airway can prevent or treat some forms of upper airway obstruction and improve oxygenation and ventilation.

Oropharyngeal vs. Nasopharyngeal Airways

Oropharyngeal airways are used to maintain airway patency in unconscious patients without a gag reflex who are having difficulty maintaining an adequate airway. The most common cause of airway obstruction in children is obstruction by the tongue, which can be prevented with the use of an oropharyngeal airway. A nasopharyngeal airway is an excellent choice for patients who are semi-conscious with an intact gag reflex; patients whose jaws are clenched, including those who are actively seizing;

and patients exhibiting snoring respirations. There are very specific contraindications to the use of each of the airway adjuncts.

Contraindications

Contraindications to the use of an airway adjunct in pediatric patients include the following:

- *Presence of a gag reflex.* Oropharyngeal airways should never be placed in patients with an intact gag reflex. Doing so may result in vomiting and aspiration. This type of airway adjunct should be used in unconscious patients only if it is required for airway patency. A nasopharyngeal airway may be a better choice when the patient's gag reflex is intact.

- *Suspected foreign body airway obstruction.* When the presence of a foreign body is known or suspected, attempts to place an oropharyngeal or nasopharyngeal airway should be avoided as it may push the object further into the airway, leading to irreversible airway obstruction.

- *Ingestion of a caustic or petroleum-based product.* When ingestion of a caustic or petroleum-based product is suspected, insertion of an oropharyngeal airway should not be attempted as it may stimulate the gag reflex resulting in vomiting and aspiration of gastric contents that can damage airway tissues. A nasopharyngeal airway is less likely to stimulate the gag reflex and therefore should be used.

- *Nasal or facial trauma or basilar skull fracture.* Trauma patients with a suspected basilar skull fracture or severe nasofacial trauma may have a fracture through the cribriform plate. A nasopharyngeal airway should not be placed as it may penetrate through this area, enter the cranial vault, and damage the brain **(Figure 4-2)**.

- *Bleeding disorders.* Patients with known bleeding disorders, such as hemophilia, should never have a nasopharyngeal airway inserted because of the risk of damage to the dense vascular bed in the nose leading to severe epistaxis (bleeding from the nose) **(Figure 4-3)**.

- *Age less than 1 year.* Age less than one year is a relative contraindication for placement of a nasopharyngeal airway. Young infants have prominent adenoids that can be injured with nasopharyngeal placement. Also, the lumen of the nasopharyngeal airway is so small in sizes appropriate for infants that it can easily be obstructed with secretions. Placing a nasopharyngeal airway in infants may remain an option if other airway opening techniques are not successful.

Positioning the Patient and Opening the Airway

Trauma Patients

video The steps for positioning the patient and opening the airway are described below.

1. Place the patient supine on a firm, flat surface, using spinal precautions. When spinal trauma is suspected, make sure to maintain the head and neck in a neutral, midline position.

2. You may place a small towel under the shoulders of any infant or young child whose large occiput prevents neutral positioning; an alternative is to use a commercially available spinal board with an occipital cutout. Placement of a towel under the shoulders is a two-person maneuver when a spinal injury is suspected; one person holds the head and neck steady in the midline position while the other places the towel under the shoulders.

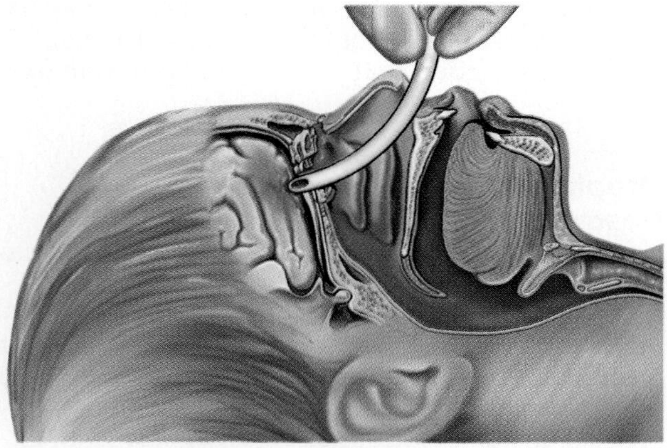

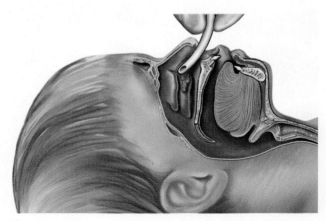

Figure 4-2 Do not use a nasopharyngeal airway in patients with facial fractures as the nasopharyngeal airway could penetrate the cribriform plate, damaging the brain.

Figure 4-3 Do not use a nasopharyngeal airway in patients with bleeding disorders, such as hemophilia, because severe bleeding can result.

3. Use the jaw-thrust maneuver to open the airway (Figure 4-4) for trauma patients. To perform a jaw thrust, place two to three fingers at the angle of the jaw on each side of the mandible. Without moving the neck or head, move the jaw forward.

   The head tilt-chin lift maneuver (Figure 4-5) is used for medical patients but is not appropriate for trauma patients because the maneuver is more likely to result in movement of the cervical spine. At no time should the head or neck be flexed or hyperextended; these positions may cause airway obstruction or spinal injury.

4. Reassess patency of airway.
5. Assess air movement.
6. Evaluate the patient's need for assisted ventilation.

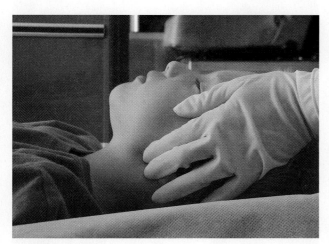

Figure 4-4 Jaw-thrust maneuver.

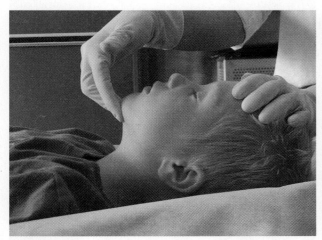

Figure 4-5 Head tilt-chin lift maneuver.

Medical Patients

For medical patients, the prehospital provider has the option to use a jaw-thrust maneuver as previously described, or the head tilt-chin lift maneuver as described below.

1. Place one hand on the forehead and while maintaining a neutral position, gently guide the head into a slight sniffing position.
2. Using the fingers of your other hand, place them on the bony portion of the mandible, at the undersurface of the chin, and lift up until the neutral sniffing position has been reached.
3. Reassess patency of airway.
4. Assess air movement.
5. Evaluate patient's need for assisted ventilation.

Measuring and Inserting Airway Adjuncts

Oropharyngeal Airway

The first step in oropharyngeal airway insertion is determining the correct size oropharyngeal airway. The size can be determined in two ways: (1) Use anatomic landmarks; and (2) use the length-based resuscitation tape.

To measure the correct size of an oropharyngeal airway using anatomic landmarks, place the airway next to the patient's face with the flange at the level of the central incisors (front teeth) and the bite block parallel to the hard palate. The tip of the appropriate size airway should reach the angle of the jaw (Figure 4-6). If the oropharyngeal airway is too small, the tongue may be pushed back into the pharynx obstructing the airway. If the airway is too large, it may obstruct the larynx.

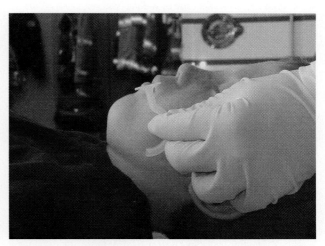

Figure 4-6 Place the oropharyngeal airway next to the patient's face with the flange at the level of the central incisors (front teeth) and the bite block parallel to the hard palate. The tip of the appropriate size airway should reach the angle of the jaw.

To use a length-based resuscitation tape or chart (Figure 4-7), find the correct size of airway by determining the length of the child, which correlates with weight and equipment sizes as discussed in Chapter 2.

Although the length-based resuscitation tape can be useful in determining the size of an oropharyngeal airway, it may be simpler to manually measure the device against the face of the child.

Insertion

Open the mouth by applying pressure on the patient's chin with your thumb. Use a tongue blade to depress the tongue, and insert the airway directly over the tongue until the flange is resting on the lips (Figure 4-8). This method does not require rotation of the airway during insertion. If a tongue blade is not available, point the oropharyngeal airway tip toward the roof of the mouth making sure not to injure the palate. Using the curved portion of the airway to depress the tongue (Figure 4-9A), rotate the airway 180° into position until the flange is resting against the lips (Figure 4-9B and 9C).

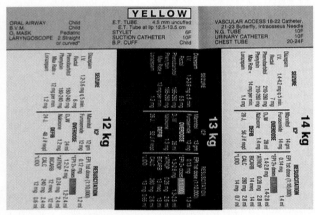

Figure 4-7 Length-based resuscitation tape with multicolored sections showing correct equipment size by weight.

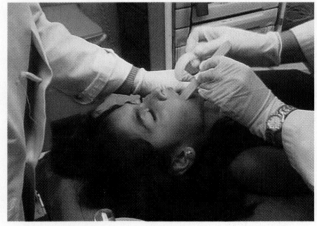

Figure 4-8 Insert the oropharyngeal airway directly over the tongue until the flange is resting on the lips.

Check the position of the airway by observing for adequate chest rise and by listening for air movement.

Nasopharyngeal Airway

Two measurements are necessary to select the appropriate size of nasopharyngeal airway for children over 1 year of age: The diameter and the length.

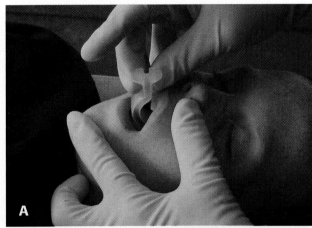

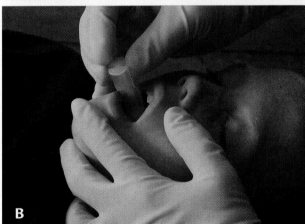

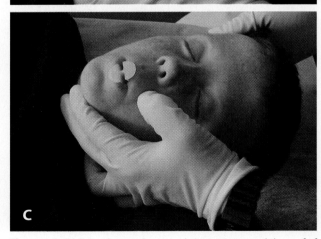

Figure 4-9 (A) Point the oropharyngeal airway tip toward the roof of the mouth making sure not to injure the palate. (B) Rotate the oropharyngeal airway 180° into position. (C) The flange of the oropharyngeal airway is resting against the lips.

Diameter

Use an airway with an outer diameter that is slightly smaller than the diameter of the nostril (Figure 4-10). An alternative method is to choose an airway with an outer diameter that is equal to the diameter of the child's little fingernail.

Length

Place the flange of the nasopharyngeal airway at the tip of the patient's nose. The tip of the airway should reach the <u>tragus</u> of the ear (Figure 4-11). If the nasopharyngeal airway has an adjustable flange, move it up or down until the length is exact.

Insertion

Once you have selected the correct size of nasopharyngeal airway, apply water-soluble lubricant to assist insertion. To place the airway in the right nostril, insert it with the bevel facing the septum while advancing the airway along the floor of the nasal cavity. Advance the airway until the flange is seated against the outside of the nostril (Figure 4-12). Note that on the right nostril, with the bevel of the nasopharyngeal airway pointed toward the septum, the curve of the nasopharyngeal airway matches the natural curve of the <u>nasopharynx</u> and can be advanced along the floor of the nasal cavity without the need to rotate it (Figure 4-13). The tip of the nasopharyngeal airway should be in the nasopharynx and there should be no blanching of the nostril. Blanching of the nostril indicates circulatory compromise of the nostril caused by a nasopharyngeal airway that is too large.

If you choose to place the airway in the left nostril, insert the airway with the tip of the airway pointing

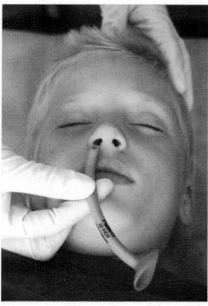

Figure 4-10 Use a nasopharyngeal airway with an outer diameter that is slightly smaller than the diameter of the nostril.

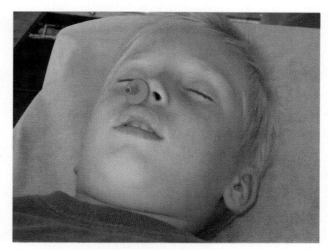

Figure 4-12 Advance the nasopharyngeal airway until the flange is seated against the outside of the nostril.

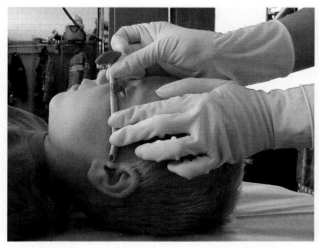

Figure 4-11 The proper length of the nasopharyngeal airway is measured by placing the flange of the nasopharyngeal airway at the tip of the patient's nose, then the tip of the airway should reach the tragus of the ear.

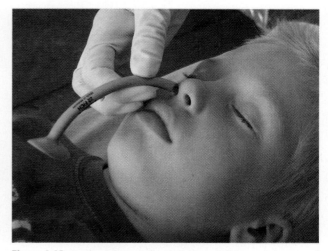

Figure 4-13 On the right nostril, with the bevel of the nasopharyngeal airway pointed toward the septum, the curve of the nasopharyngeal airway matches the natural curve of the nasopharynx.

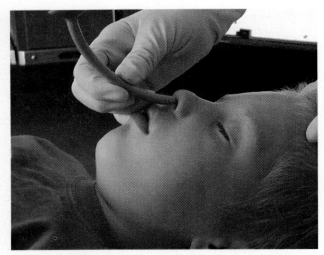

Figure 4-14 On the left nostril, with the bevel of the nasopharyngeal airway pointed toward the septum, the curve of the nasopharyngeal airway will be upside down as compared to the floor of the nasal cavity.

upward, which will allow the bevel to face the septum (Figure 4-14). Advance the airway with the tip directed along the floor of the nasal cavity until resistance is met (approximately 1–2 cm), then rotate the airway 180° into position. Reassess airway patency by listening for air movement and observing for chest rise.

TRICKS
of the Trade

To maximize airway opening in a child lying supine, place a small towel under the child's shoulders, elevating the shoulders slightly. Make sure the child's head is held midline and is not allowed to move in any direction on the neck when spinal trauma is suspected. Correct positioning prevents folds of soft tissue in the short neck of an infant or young child from obstructing the airway.

Problem Solving

If the patient's jaws are clenched, preventing insertion of an oropharyngeal airway, consider using a nasopharyngeal airway instead.

If the effectiveness of a nasopharyngeal airway seems to be diminishing, assess for obstruction of the lumen with mucus, blood, emesis, or soft tissue. Consider suctioning and if this does not improve the situation, remove the nasopharyngeal airway.

If you notice blanching of the nostril after insertion, remove the nasopharyngeal airway, and replace it with one that has a smaller diameter.

Procedure Step-by-Step

video The steps for using an airway adjunct are described below and in **Skill Drill 4-1**. Assess the PAT and ABCDEs and determine if there is an indication for airway positioning or use of an airway adjunct to maintain airway patency.

1. Position the patient.
   Open the airway.
   - Use the jaw-thrust maneuver for trauma patients.
   - Use the head tilt-chin lift or jaw-thrust maneuver for medical patients.

Depending on whether or not the patient has an intact gag reflex, proceed to either Step 2 (no gag reflex) or Step 4 (intact gag reflex).
Use an oropharyngeal airway for patients who do not have an intact gag reflex.

2. Select the correct size. Use anatomic landmarks (front teeth or upper gum line, angle of the jaw). Use the length-based resuscitation tape.

3. Insert the oropharyngeal airway.
   - Use a tongue blade to depress the tongue and make room for airway insertion, or
   - Use the upside-down rotation method.
   - Reassess airway patency and observe for chest rise.

Use a nasopharyngeal airway for patients with an intact gag reflex.

4. Select the correct size of nasopharyngeal airway (measure from the tip of nose to the tragus of the ear). Move the flange up and down as needed to achieve the correct length. Lubricate the nasopharyngeal airway.

5. Right nostril insertion:
   - Bevel toward septum
   - No need to rotate
   - Advance until the flange is seated against the outside of the nostril.

6. Left nostril insertion:
   - Bevel toward septum (upside down)
   - Insert until resistance is met.
   - Rotate the airway 180° into position with the flange seated against the outside of nostril.

7. Reassess airway patency.

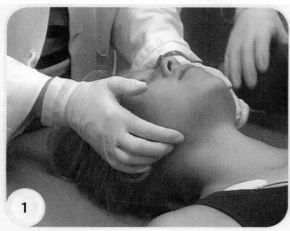

1

Position the patient.

Open the airway (jaw-thrust maneuver for trauma patients; head tilt-chin lift or jaw-thrust maneuver for medical patients).

Depending on whether or not the patient has an intact gag reflex, proceed to either Step 2 (no gag reflex) or Step 4 (intact gag reflex).

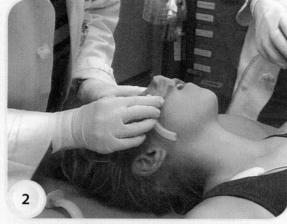

2

For patients with no gag reflex, select the correct size oropharyngeal airway.

Use anatomic landmarks (front teeth or upper gum line, angle of the jaw).

Use the length-based resuscitation tape.

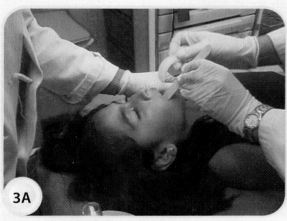

3A

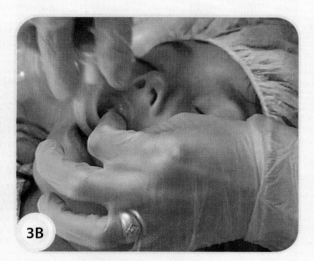

3B

Insert the oropharyngeal airway.

- Use a tongue blade to depress the tongue and make room for airway insertion (**A**), or
- Use the upside-down rotation method (**B**).
- Reassess airway patency and observe for chest rise.

Continued

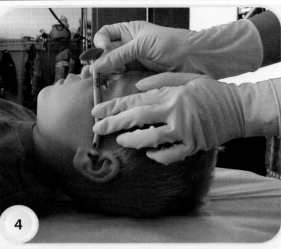

4

For patients with an intact gag reflex, select the correct size nasopharyngeal airway (measure from the tip of nose to the tragus of the ear). Move the flange up and down as needed to achieve the correct length. Lubricate the nasopharyngeal airway.

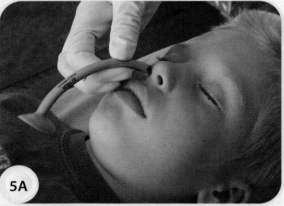

5A

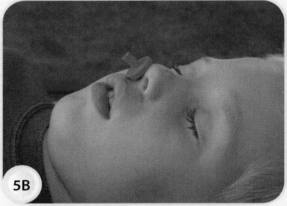

5B

Right nostril insertion: Bevel toward septum, no need to rotate (**A**). Advance until the flange is seated against the outside of the nostril (**B**).

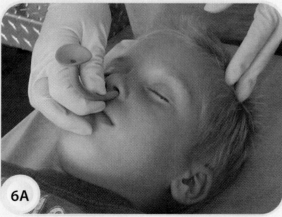

6A

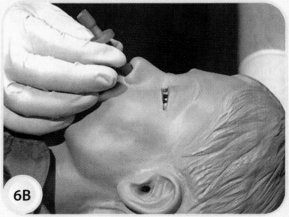

6B

Left nostril insertion: Bevel toward septum (upside down) (**A**). Insert until resistance is met. Rotate the airway 180° into position with the flange seated against the outside of nostril (**B**).

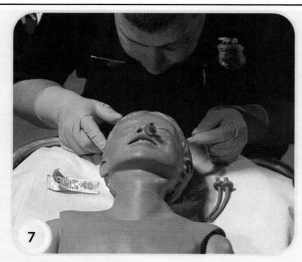

7

Reassess airway patency.

Complications

Complications of using an airway adjunct in a pediatric patient include the following:

- Vomiting
- Obstruction of the airway
- Laceration of soft tissue
- Laceration of the palate
- Vagal stimulation
- Gastric distention
- Laryngospasm
- Laceration of adenoidal tissue or nasal mucosa
- Epistaxis
- Potential for increased intracranial pressure

Prevention of Complications

You can prevent vomiting on insertion of an oropharyngeal airway by making sure the patient does not have an intact gag reflex prior to insertion. Problems such as airway obstruction by the tongue can be prevented by carefully measuring for the correct size of oropharyngeal airway. The tongue can be pushed against the posterior pharynx when too small an airway is used. When too large an oropharyngeal airway is used, obstruction can be caused by the airway itself. Use of good technique on insertion will minimize the risk of trauma to soft tissues in the mouth.

Most providers avoid insertion of nasopharyngeal airways in infants because mucus, blood, vomitus, or the soft tissues of the pharynx can obstruct the tiny internal diameter of the airway. Be careful to choose the correct size of nasopharyngeal airway and to follow the proper steps for insertion. If you insert a nasopharyngeal airway that is too long, you can cause laryngospasm and vomiting in responsive patients. Insertion of a nasopharyngeal airway in a patient with head trauma may cause increased intracranial pressure. This is a theoretical concern as studies have been done only using nasal suctioning of the airway. When you suspect a basilar skull fracture, do not place a nasal airway as there is a concern that the nasopharyngeal airway may perforate the cranial vault through the fracture site and enter the brain. Finally, proper sizing and correct insertion technique can help to avert laceration of adenoidal tissue or the nasal mucosa leading to epistaxis or bleeding into the nasopharynx.

Conclusions

After positioning the patient and opening the airway, continue to reassess the patient. If there is adequate chest rise initially, and the patient has no chest rise after placement of an oropharyngeal airway, re-evaluate the sizing and placement of the oropharyngeal airway, and consider the possibility of foreign body obstruction.

Scenario Review

You have responded to an intersection where you found a 10-year-old boy who was hit by a truck as he rode his bike across the street. Upon arrival, you noted that the boy was unresponsive with a high-pitched cry. There was a large laceration on his forehead.

1. *What are your initial assessment priorities?*

Your first priority is assessment of the PAT and the ABCDEs. The airway is open, there are no abnormal airway sounds, and the boy has spontaneous respirations at a rate of 6 breaths/min with decreased tidal volume. His skin color is pale and peripheral pulses are present with a rate of 80. He is unconscious, unresponsive to voice or painful stimuli, and has signs of head trauma.

2. *What are your initial treatment priorities?*

Place him in the supine position while maintaining spinal stabilization. Open the airway using a jaw-thrust maneuver and reassess adequacy of ventilation. There is no improvement in rate or tidal volume after you have opened the airway.

3. *Would you consider placing an airway adjunct in this patient?*

Yes, this patient has altered level of consciousness and signs of head trauma, thus an oropharyngeal airway would be the best choice to maintain an open airway. After you place the oropharyngeal airway and administer 100% oxygen by nonrebreather mask, his color, respiratory rate and tidal volume improve. His level of consciousness also improves, the patient begins to gag, and you remove the oropharyngeal airway. You decide to transport him rapidly to the nearest appropriate receiving facility.

Quick Quiz

1. *To ensure that the airway is open in an infant or child, you would:*
   A. Make sure the neck is flexed forward.
   B. Make sure the head is hyperextended on the neck.
   C. Make sure the head is in neutral midline position.
   D. Place a small towel under the infant's head.

2. *Indications for the use of a nasopharyngeal airway include:*
   A. Nasofacial trauma.
   B. Bleeding disorders.
   C. Suspected basilar skull fracture.
   D. Actively seizing patients.
   E. Age less than 1 year.

3. *An improperly sized oropharyngeal airway may:*
   A. Push the tongue into the posterior pharynx, obstructing the airway.
   B. Enter the esophagus.
   C. Cause lacerations of the tongue.
   D. Be trimmed to proper length with a scalpel or scissors.

4. *When placing a nasopharyngeal airway in the right nostril:*
   A. Rotate 180° degrees after inserting approximately one inch.
   B. Add an oropharyngeal airway to ensure the airway is open prior to nasopharyngeal airway insertion.
   C. Place bevel facing the septum as it enters the nostril.
   D. Nasopharyngeal airways should not be placed in the right nostril.
   E. The airway should not be lubricated prior to insertion.

Glossary

cribriform plate   Perforated structure separating the nasal airway passage from the brain.

epistaxis   Bleeding from the nose.

hard palate   The hard portion of the roof of the mouth, separating the mouth from the nasal cavity.

laryngospasm   A spasm of the laryngeal muscles.

nasopharynx   The part of the pharynx situated above the soft palate and behind the nose.

palate   The horizontal structure separating the mouth and the nasal cavity; the roof of the mouth.

patency   The state of being freely open.

patent   Open and unobstructed.

pharynx   Passageway for air (from nasal cavity to larynx) and food (from mouth to esophagus).

tragus   Cartilaginous projection in front of the exterior meatus of the ear.

vagal   Pertaining to the vagus nerve and cholinergic nervous system.

Selected References

1. American Academy of Pediatrics. *Pediatric Education for Prehospital Professionals.* Sudbury, Mass: Jones and Bartlett Publishers; 2000.

2. American Heart Association. Guidelines 2000 for cardiopulmonary resuscitation and emergency cardiovascular care. *Circulation.* 2000;102:8.

3. Foltin G, Tunik M, Cooper A, et al. *Teaching Resource for Instructors in Prehospital Pediatrics (EMT-Basic).* New York: Maternal and Child Health Bureau; 1998.

4. Hazinski MF, Zaritsky AL, Nadkarni VM (eds), et al. *PALS Provider Manual.* Dallas: American Heart Association; 2000;91–126.

5. Seidel, JS, Henderson, DP. *Prehospital Care of Pediatric Emergencies.* 2nd ed. Sudbury, Mass: Jones and Bartlett Publishers; 1997;209–214.

End of Chapter Activities

Technology Resources

Online Course

Anatomy Review

Online Glossary

Web Links

Online Quiz

Scenarios

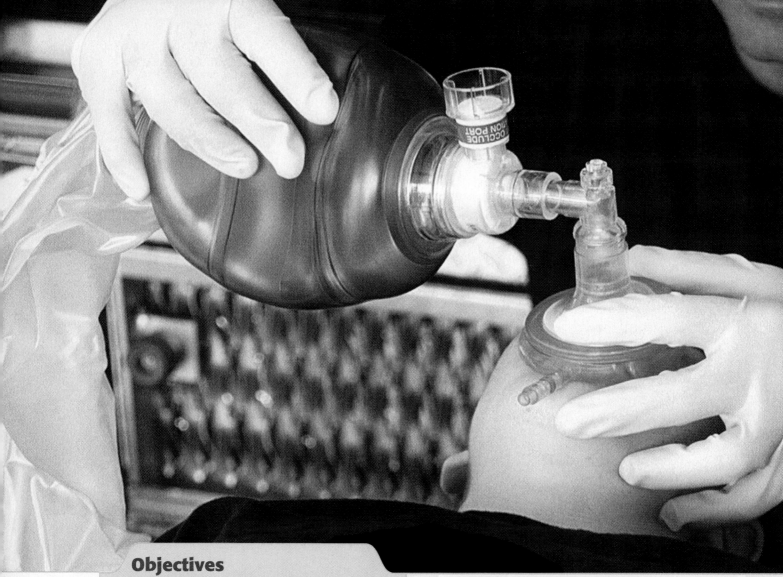

Objectives

1 List the indications and contraindications in use of bag-mask ventilation.

2 Determine the correct size mask and manual resuscitator for bag-mask ventilation.

3 Outline the procedure for bag-mask ventilation using one-handed and two-handed techniques.

4 Identify complications in using bag-mask ventilation, then determine corrective measures.

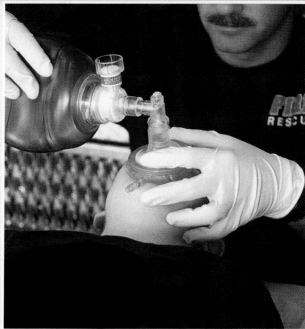

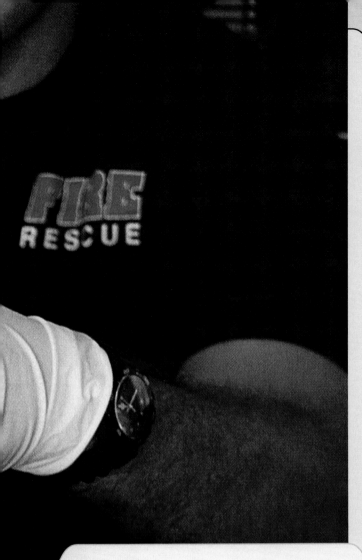

CHAPTER 5

Bag-Mask Ventilation

Scenario

You are called to the scene of a 7-year-old boy with a seizure. Upon arrival you note that the child is pale, there are frothy secretions at the lips, and the child is seizing with rhythmic movements of all extremities. Your priorities are to maintain oxygenation and ventilation and to stop the seizure.

You position the child's head and suction the mouth before providing 15L oxygen by nonrebreather mask. A cardiac monitor and pulse oximeter are placed. The seizure stops, but the patient's color is now cyanotic and the heart rate drops to 80 beats per minute; the pulse oximeter reads 89%. Placement of a nasopharyngeal airway does not improve oxygenation or ventilation.

1. *What are your management priorities now?*

2. *How would you assess the adequacy of your interventions?*

Think about these questions and this case as you read on. We will return to this scenario at the end of the chapter.

57

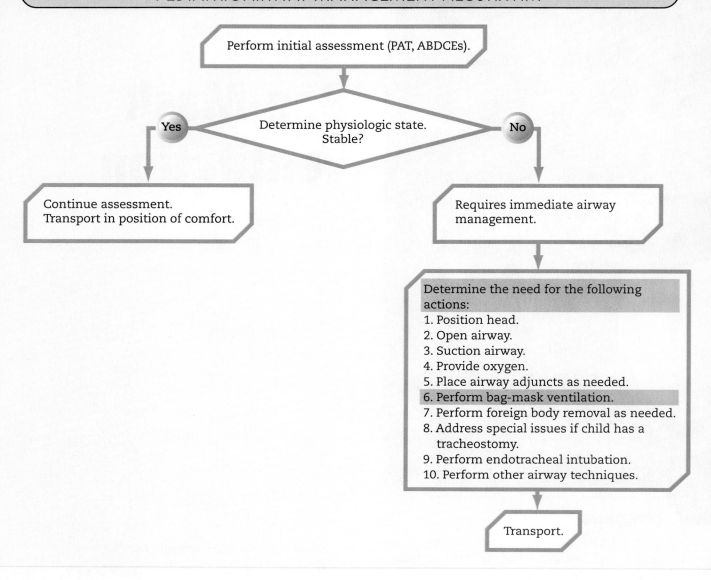

Perform initial assessment (PAT, ABDCEs).

Yes ← Determine physiologic state. Stable? → **No**

Continue assessment.
Transport in position of comfort.

Requires immediate airway management.

Determine the need for the following actions:
1. Position head.
2. Open airway.
3. Suction airway.
4. Provide oxygen.
5. Place airway adjuncts as needed.
6. Perform bag-mask ventilation.
7. Perform foreign body removal as needed.
8. Address special issues if child has a tracheostomy.
9. Perform endotracheal intubation.
10. Perform other airway techniques.

Transport.

Introduction

The skill of bag-mask ventilation is the linchpin of airway management for the pediatric patient. It is the procedure performed initially in virtually all cases of respiratory failure requiring support of ventilation. It is the rescue method when other forms of airway management, such as endotracheal intubation, fail.

Anatomical Considerations

video Anatomical differences in children versus adults relevant to performance of bag-mask ventilation include:

- Proportionately larger occiput
- Relatively larger tongue
- Less mature chest and abdominal musculature

Anatomical differences in adults and children are important to consider when performing bag-mask ventilation. The large occiput in young children may cause the head to flex on the neck, which may cause airway obstruction. Placement of a small towel under the shoulders helps to level the plane of the pediatric airway. The large size of the tongue, relative to the mouth, in children may lead to airway obstruction as the tongue falls back into the back of the oropharynx; therefore, it is important to position the head in the midline in sniffing position with the head slightly extended on the neck and to use airway opening maneuvers or adjuncts to keep the airway open during the procedure. Correct hand placement on the jaw will facilitate good head position and avoidance of pressure on the <u>submental area</u> (the area beneath the chin) will ensure that the tongue is not pushed back into the oropharynx during bag-mask ventilation. Finally,

Where's the Evidence?

Bag-Mask Ventilation

The evidence for ventilation technique and the effectiveness of bag-mask ventilation in the prehospital setting comes mainly from experience in the operating room, simulated ventilation models, and a large controlled trial of bag-mask ventilation and endotracheal intubation.

Wenzel and colleagues studied 80 adult patients in respiratory arrest prior to elective intubation in the operating room. These patients were randomized to receive lower ventilatory volumes (bag-mask device or self-inflating manual resuscitator 750 ml) versus higher ventilatory volumes (bag-mask device or self-inflating manual resuscitator 1,500 ml). The authors found that the oxygen saturation of the two groups was comparable. They also found that the end-tidal carbon dioxide was greater in the group receiving the smaller volumes and that no patient in this group had gastric insufflation (distention) compared to four patients (10%) in the higher volume group. The authors concluded that administering smaller tidal volumes in patients with respiratory arrest achieves good oxygenation and prevents gastric insufflation.

Melker and Banner found in a simulated ventilation model that increasing the inspiratory time also reduced gastric insufflation.

Moynihan and colleagues evaluated the use of cricoid pressure (the Sellick maneuver) in preventing gastric insufflation in infants and children. They found that appropriately applied cricoid pressure was 100% effective in preventing gastric insufflation into the stomachs of infants and children ages 2 weeks to 8 years.

Kanter, in a study of pediatric resident physicians, nurses, and respiratory therapists, found that ventilation of a 4-kg manikin using a manual resus-citator could be achieved with reasonable success. The investigators also found that many of the health care professionals used excessive volumes of air at too high a pressure when ventilating this simulated pediatric patient.

Gausche and colleagues, using a technique to reduce the likelihood that paramedic rescuers would use excessive pressures and volumes with bag-mask ventilation ("squeeze, release, release"), found that outcomes of children treated with bag-mask ventilation were as good or better than outcomes of children treated with endotracheal intubation in the prehospital setting. This technique requires the rescuer to say "squeeze" as the bag of the manual resuscitator is being squeezed. By saying "squeeze" the inspiratory time for assisted ventilation is slightly increased. During the squeeze phase the rescuer looks for the initiation of chest rise—when that occurs, the bag is released so that excessive volume will not be delivered. The rescuer then states "release, release" as the patient is allowed to passively exhale. When the "squeeze, release, release" technique is utilized, it helps to calm the rescuer while achieving adequate ventilation and oxygenation for the patient.

1. Gausche M, Lewis RJ, Stratton SJ. Effect of out-of-hospital pediatric endotracheal intubation on survival and neurological outcome: A controlled clinical trial. *JAMA*. 2000;283:6:783–790.
2. Kantor RK. Evaluation of mask-bag ventilation in resuscitation of infants. *AJDC*. 1987;141:761–763.
3. Melker RJ, Banner MJ. Ventilation during CPR: Two-rescuer standard reappraisal. *Ann Emerg Med*. 1985;14:397–402.
4. Moynihan RJ, Brock-Utne JG, Archer JH, et al. The effect of cricoid pressure on preventing gastric insufflation in infants and children. *Anesthesiology*. 1993 Apr;78(4):652–656.
5. Wenzel V, Keller C, Idris AH, et al. Effects of smaller tidal volumes during basic life support ventilation in patients with respiratory arrest: Good ventilation, less risk? *Resuscitation*. 1999;43:25–29.

the less mature chest and abdominal musculature result in more dependence on diaphragmatic excursion (movement) to achieve adequate ventilation. Gastric insufflation that may occur with rescue ventilation can prevent adequate diaphragmatic movement and lead to hypoventilation. This is why it is key to not deliver too much air with each ventilation when performing bag-mask ventilation. It is also important to achieve an adequate seal on the mask. It can be difficult even for an experienced practitioner to provide a perfect seal with one hand, especially in adolescents or adults. Careful attention to maintaining the seal and, in selected patients, use of a two-hand seal with an assistant squeezing the bag, can prevent air leakage.

Indications

Indications for bag-mask ventilation in pediatric patients include the following:
- Respiratory failure
- Respiratory arrest
- Cardiopulmonary failure

Bag-mask ventilation is indicated for initial support of ventilation and oxygenation when compensatory mechanisms fail and the patient is in respiratory failure. It is important to realize that in some situations positioning of the head, suctioning, adding an airway adjunct, or providing supplemental oxygen can result in improvement of the patient's condition to a point where assisted ventilation is not needed. If these maneuvers are not successful in treating the patient with respiratory failure, or if the patient is in respiratory arrest or cardiopulmonary failure, then bag-mask ventilation should begin without delay.

Contraindications

Contraindications to performing bag-mask ventilation in pediatric patients include the following:
- Stable respiratory status
- Respiratory distress with clinical signs of adequate ventilation and oxygenation

Patients with a stable respiratory status or those patients with signs of adequate oxygenation and ventilation should not receive bag-mask ventilation as the technique may result in gastric insufflation, vomiting, or aspiration.

Other problems that may complicate use of a bag-mask device include:
- Facial trauma, including open cheek lacerations, fractures of the mandible, and large, open facial wounds
- Facial burns
- Severe bronchospasm with limited chest excursion
- Airway obstruction
- Neck instability

Procedure Step-by-Step

video The first step in the performance of any procedure is the assessment of the need for the intervention. Assess the infant or child using the PAT and ABCDEs. If the child is in respiratory or cardiopulmonary failure, begin the procedure.

Gather your equipment. This will need to be done quickly as the patient is in immediate need of assisted ventilation. Storage of pediatric-sized equipment in a handy storage bag that is clearly marked can facilitate locating the proper equipment. This equipment will include an oxygen tank; oxygen tubing; pediatric bag-mask device (also called a manual resuscitator); various sizes of masks, gloves, and other personal protective equipment; various sizes of airway adjuncts; and a suction device.

Be sure that the oxygen tubing from the mask is attached to the oxygen tank and the tank is turned on to deliver 15L of oxygen per minute.

Measure the mask. This can be done simply by placing the mask on the patient's face; the correct size mask will measure from the bridge of the nose to the cleft of the chin (Figure 5-1). Avoid compression of the eyes as this can cause a vagal response in the child, resulting in slowing of the heart rate. Once you have chosen the correct size mask, attach it to the end of the elbow adapter on the manual resuscitator.

Form a "C" with your thumb and index finger (Figure 5-2). Place the mask back on the patient's face and wrap your thumb around the mask at the end of the mask that lies on the bridge of the nose; place your index finger around the portion of the mask over the chin. Place your long, ring, and small fingers along the angle of the jaw forming an "E" (Figure 5-3). Bag-mask ventilation is as "EC" as 1-2-3. This technique is called the EC-clamp. Use your "E" fingers to gently pull the chin into the mask. Do not place your fingers in the soft tissue under the chin as pressure in this area can compress the airway or cause the tongue to fall back against the posterior pharynx (back of the mouth), leading to airway obstruction.

Instruct your colleague to place gentle cricoid pressure as you prepare to ventilate the patient. This may decrease the amount of air that enters the stomach by compressing the esophagus against the spine. Too much cricoid pressure can obstruct the airway.

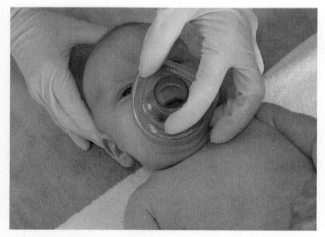

Figure 5-1 Measure the mask from the bridge of the nose to the cleft of the chin.

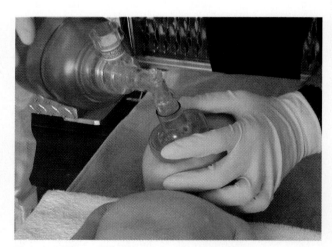

Figure 5-2 Form a "C" with your thumb and index finger.

Begin to ventilate the patient by squeezing the bag. The rescuer will say "squeeze" as the bag is being squeezed (Figure 5-4). Say "squeeze" over 1 to 1.5 seconds. This increased inspiratory time decreases gastric insufflation. Squeeze the bag or manual resuscitator only until chest rise is begun. It is important to note that in infants and young children, the lower chest and upper abdomen rise with appropriate ventilation. The stomach area should not increase in size. You don't need to inflate the chest fully—by doing so, additional air will inflate the stomach. Once you see the chest rise, begin releasing the bag and say "release, release." This allows time for exhalation. The rescuer says "squeeze, release, release" to complete the whole sequence. The respiratory rate should approach 40 breaths/min for a neonate, 20–30 breaths/min for an infant, and 20 breaths/min for a child. Excessive ventilation rates and pressure delivered leads to complications such as gastric insufflation, vomiting, and aspiration. Reassess the patient for improved color, heart rate, and overall clinical status.

Bag-mask ventilation can be summarized into the following steps and is shown in **Skill Drill 5-1**.

1. Position the head.
2. Measure the mask from the bridge of the nose to the cleft of the chin. Attach the bag-mask device, which should already be connected to oxygen.
3. Perform the EC-clamp.
4. Pull the chin into the mask.
5. Say "squeeze, release, release" while doing the same.
6. Assess for chest rise.

7. Consider using the two-rescuer technique.
   Consider using an airway adjunct if there is no chest rise.
   Consider the possibility of foreign body airway obstruction if there is no chest rise.
   Check for signs of improvement.

TRICKS
of the Trade

Performing successful bag-mask ventilation requires patience and good technique. The first steps of measuring the mask and placing it on the face using the "EC-clamp" are quite important. Too much downward pressure placed on the mask can result in the head flexing forward onto the neck and can cause partial or complete occlusion of the airway. If this occurs, reposition the head by placing a towel under the shoulders for small children or infants or by extending the head.

Providers are often quite anxious when faced with management of a child's airway and providing assisted ventilation. Many ventilate the patient at their own personal pulse rate. Don't do this; remain calm. Saying "squeeze, release, release" helps to slow ventilation rates and reduces anxiety in the provider. Also, the amount of volume that is delivered is smaller than you think. In a neonate weighing 3 kg, the amount of air that will be needed to cause the chest to rise is about 30 ml or 2 tablespoons of air; in a 1-year-old this amount is about 7 tablespoons of air. This is why vigorously squeezing the bag and delivering high volumes of air leads to complications; the lungs fill quickly and all the air goes into the stomach. Gently squeeze the bag with just the right pressure and volume—no more!—to cause the chest to rise.

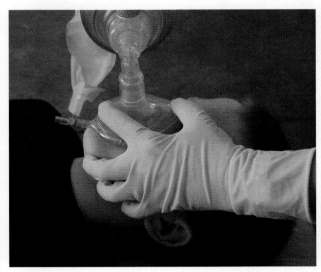

Figure 5-3 Place your long, ring, and small fingers along the angle of the jaw, forming an "E" as part of the EC-clamp.

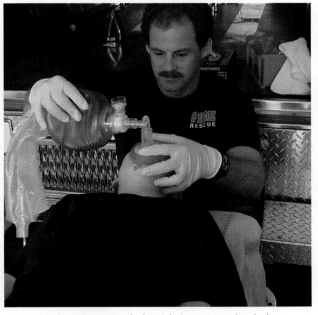

Figure 5-4 Say "squeeze" as the bag is being squeezed and release once chest rise is initiated.

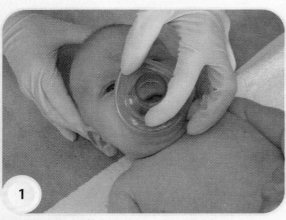

1

Position the head.

Measure the mask from the bridge of the nose to the cleft of the chin.

Attach the bag-mask device, which should already be connected to oxygen.

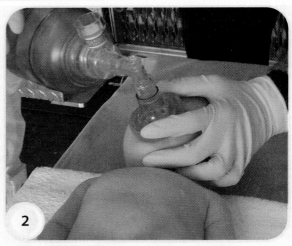

2

Perform the EC-clamp.

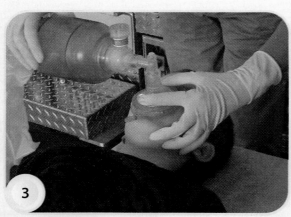

3

Pull the chin into the mask.

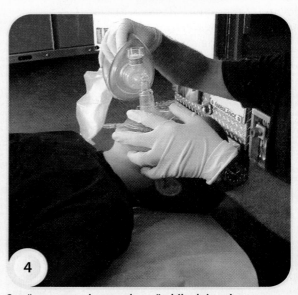

4

Say "squeeze, release, release" while doing the same.

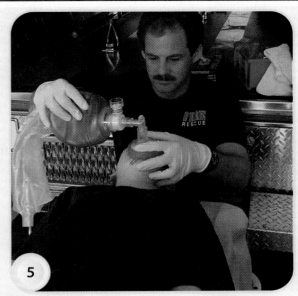

5

Assess for chest rise.

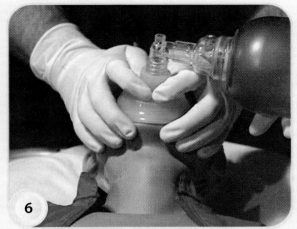

6

Consider using the two-rescuer technique.

Consider using an airway adjunct if there is no chest rise.

Consider the possibility of foreign body airway obstruction if there is no chest rise.

Check for signs of improvement.

Complications

Complications that can result during bag-mask ventilation include:

- Gastric insufflation
- Vomiting
- Aspiration
- Hypoxia
- Barotrauma

Each of these complications can be minimized if the correct technique is used. Correctly sizing the mask and ensuring that the bag-device (manual resuscitator) is connected to 100% oxygen will help to reduce the risk of hypoxia. Patients can be ventilated with this technique for hours while maintaining an oxygen saturation of 98–100%. In a prehospital study in Los Angeles and Orange Counties, California, patients receiving bag-mask ventilation had an average oxygen saturation of 98% on arrival in the emergency department; one patient was ventilated by this technique for 55 minutes. Eighty-five percent of the children could be bag-mask ventilated with one rescuer; in the other patients, the two-rescuer technique was preferred. Using the "squeeze, release, release" technique will reduce the volume of oxygen delivered and slow the rate of ventilation. These steps will reduce the risk of barotrauma as well as gastric insufflation, vomiting, and aspiration. Adding cricoid pressure also reduces the risk of gastric insufflation. Remember that if too much cricoid pressure is placed, the airway of the child will be obstructed and attempts at ventilation will result in no chest rise. In this case, release cricoid pressure and reassess the patient for chest rise with assisted ventilation.

If you note air freely escaping from the sides of the mask, then either the mask seal is not adequate or you are delivering too much pressure of air with each ventilation. Reposition the head and pull the chin into the mask to get a better seal. Squeeze the bag with just enough pressure to cause the lower chest to rise.

Conclusions

Bag-mask ventilation is a skill that needs to be mastered by all levels of health care providers. This airway technique will be used far more often than other techniques to provide assisted ventilation. Practicing these methods as often as is possible on manikins or in the operating room setting will assist in maintaining mastery of these techniques.

Scenario Review

You were called to the scene of a 7-year-old boy with a seizure. Upon arrival you noted that the child was pale; there were frothy secretions at the lips and the child was seizing with rhythmic movements of all extremities. Your priorities were to maintain oxygenation and ventilation and stop the seizure.

You positioned the child's head and suctioned the mouth before providing oxygen 15 L by partial nonrebreather mask. A cardiac monitor and pulse oximeter were placed. The seizure stopped, but the patient's color was cyanotic and the heart rate dropped to 80 beats per minute; the pulse oximeter read 89%. Placement of a nasopharyngeal airway did not improve oxygenation or ventilation.

1. *What are your management priorities now?*

Your priority is to begin assisted ventilation. You reposition the head and then begin bag-mask ventilation. Be sure to say "squeeze, release, release" as you are ventilating the patient. Watch for chest rise and do not deliver too much air with each breath.

2. *How would you assess the adequacy of your interventions?*

You assess for the adequacy of your intervention by looking for chest rise and improvement in the patient's clinical condition.

In this case, bag-mask ventilation results in the patient's color improving, the heart rate increases to 120 and the oxygen saturation increases to 97%. During transport the patient begins to move and fight the ventilation. Bag-mask ventilation is discontinued and the patient is placed on 15L oxygen by mask.

This scenario demonstrates the importance of the stepwise approach to airway management, the need for reassessment, and the utility of bag-mask ventilation to provide oxygenation and ventilation in the pediatric patient.

Quick Quiz

1. *Which of the following are the most important anatomical landmarks on the child for sizing a mask for bag-mask ventilation?*
   A. Tip of nose to mid-portion of the lip
   B. Between the eyes to under the chin
   C. Bridge of nose to cleft of chin
   D. Forehead to bottom of lip

2. *Which of the following statements best describes the way the provider determines if enough air has been delivered with bag-mask ventilation?*
   A. The patient's chest fully expands.
   B. Deliver enough air to cause air to escape freely out the sides of the mask.
   C. The patient's lower chest begins to rise.
   D. The lower abdomen increases in size with each ventilation.

3. *Pressure in the submental area (under the chin) with your fingers while performing bag-mask ventilation can lead to which of the following airway problems?*
   A. Upper airway obstruction
   B. Lower airway obstruction
   C. Fluid in the lungs
   D. Airway injury

4. *Which of the following methods has been shown to be effective in the prehospital management of children requiring bag-mask ventilation?*
   A. Delivering rapid, short breaths at 60 per minute.
   B. Delivering breaths with slower inspiration times and adequate volumes.
   C. Ventilating the child quickly while utilizing the entire volume of air available in the manual resuscitator.
   D. Ventilating the infant with five breaths followed by 10-second pauses to simulate periodic breathing.

Glossary

cricoid pressure   The technique of placing pressure on either side of the cricoid cartilage on the neck to prevent gastric insufflation during endotracheal intubation; also called the Sellick maneuver.

EC-clamp   A maneuver used to create an effective seal when ventilating a patient. An "E" is formed by placing the long, ring, and small fingers along the angle of the jaw. A "C" is formed by placing the thumb and index finger around the edge of the mask.

gastric insufflation   The introduction of air into the stomach, which can be a complication of ventilation; also called distention.

hypoventilation   A reduction in the amount of air that is entering the lungs, either from reduced rate and/or depth of breathing.

manual resuscitator   A type of ventilation bag. There are two types: a self-inflating bag and an anesthesia bag. In the field, the self-inflating bag is also called a bag-mask device.

Sellick maneuver The technique of placing pressure on either side of the cricoid cartilage on the neck to prevent gastric insufflation during endotracheal intubation; also called cricoid pressure.

submental area The area beneath the chin.

Selected References

1. Dieckmann RA, Brownstein D, Gausche-Hill M, eds. *Pediatric Education for Prehospital Professionals: PEPP Textbook.* Sudbury, Mass: Jones and Bartlett Publishers; 2000.

2. Gausche M, Lewis RJ, Stratton SJ, et al. Effect of out-of-hospital pediatric endotracheal intubation on survival and neurological outcome: A controlled clinical trial. JAMA. 2000;283:6:783–790.

3. Gausche-Hill M, Dieckmann RA, Brownstein D, eds. *Pediatric Education for Prehospital Professionals: PEPP Resource Manual.* Sudbury, Mass: Jones and Bartlett Publishers; 2000.

4. Kantor RK. Evaluation of bag-mask ventilation in resuscitation of infants. *AJDC.* 1987;141:761–763.

5. Melker RJ, Banner MJ. Ventilation during CPR: Two-rescuer standard reappraisal. *Ann Emerg Med.* 1985;14;397–402.

6. Moynihan RJ, Brock-Utne JG, Archer JH, et al. The effect of cricoid pressure on preventing gastric insufflation in infants and children. *Anesthesiology.* April 1993;78(4):652–656.

7. Wenzel V, Keller C, Idris AH, et al. Effects of smaller tidal volumes during basic life support ventilation in patients with respiratory arrest: Good ventilation, less risk? *Resuscitation.* 1999;43:25–29.

Technology Resources

Online Course _ _ _ _ _ _ _ _ _ _ _ _ _ _ _

Anatomy Review _ _ _ _ _ _ _ _ _ _ _ _ _

Online Glossary _ _ _ _ _ _ _ _ _ _ _ _ _

Web Links _ _ _ _ _ _ _ _ _ _ _ _ _ _ _ _ _

Online Quiz _ _ _ _ _ _ _ _ _ _ _ _ _ _ _ _

Scenarios

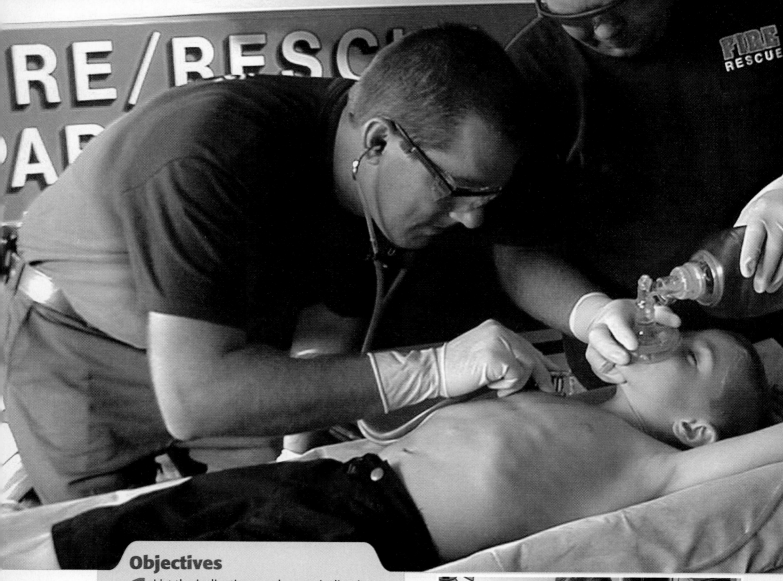

Objectives

1 List the indications and contraindications for removal of an airway foreign body.

2 Determine the need for intervention and outline the procedure for foreign body removal.

3 Identify the complications of foreign body aspiration and removal, then determine corrective measures.

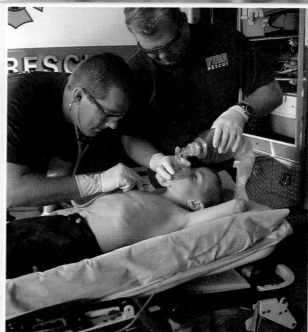

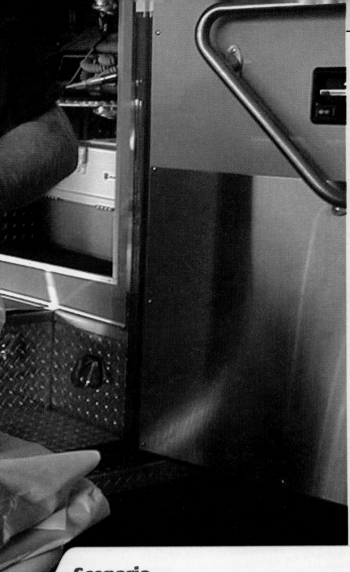

CHAPTER 6

Foreign Body Removal

Scenario

You respond in the evening to a private residence and find law enforcement personnel performing CPR on a 4-year-old boy. Your initial assessment reveals that the boy is apneic but has a palpable pulse rate of 80 beats per minute. CPR is discontinued. You attempt ventilation with a bag-mask device. You see no chest rise with ventilation.

1. *What are the possible reasons for a lack of chest rise?*

2. *What are your immediate interventions?*

Think about these questions and this case as you read on. We will return to this scenario at the end of the chapter.

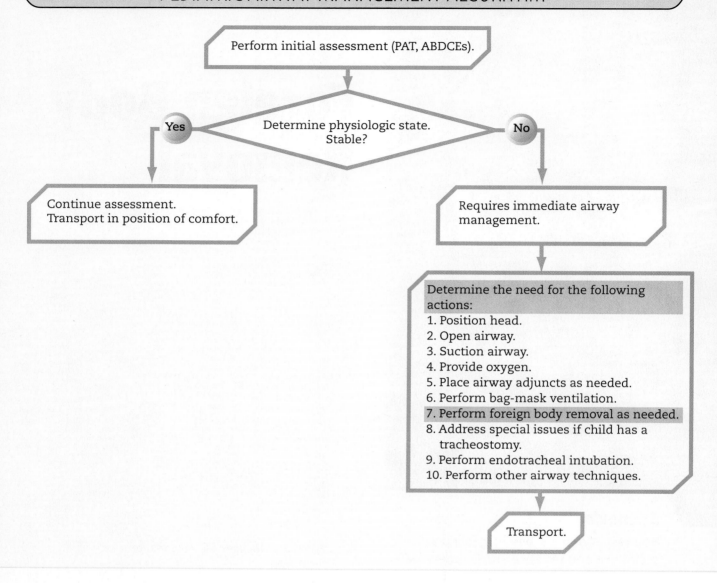

Perform initial assessment (PAT, ABDCEs).

Determine physiologic state. Stable?

Yes → Continue assessment. Transport in position of comfort.

No → Requires immediate airway management.

Determine the need for the following actions:
1. Position head.
2. Open airway.
3. Suction airway.
4. Provide oxygen.
5. Place airway adjuncts as needed.
6. Perform bag-mask ventilation.
7. Perform foreign body removal as needed.
8. Address special issues if child has a tracheostomy.
9. Perform endotracheal intubation.
10. Perform other airway techniques.

Transport.

Introduction

Few pediatric emergencies create the same sense of urgency and degree of anxiety as an airway obstruction. You may find yourself faced with an unconscious, cyanotic infant or child whom you are unable to ventilate adequately. Family and bystanders may be unaware of what led to this condition or may be unable to communicate it to those who are urgently trying to identify the cause of the obstruction and relieve it. You perform a quick assessment, intervene appropriately, and follow the proper sequence of basic life support (BLS) interventions before advanced life support (ALS) interventions.

Some objects (especially small round objects the same diameter as the airway) are difficult to grasp even when the proper equipment is available. In some cases it may take multiple attempts to remove the ob-

structing object(s) completely. In other cases bystanders' attempts to remove the object prior to your arrival may have caused bleeding, swelling, and trauma to the airway, making landmarks difficult to identify.

In these situations, understanding the anatomy and potential causes of airway obstruction can assist in creative problem solving, which may result in removing the foreign body and saving the life of the patient.

Anatomical Considerations

video Anatomical differences in children versus adults relevant to foreign body removal include:

Where's the Evidence?

Foreign Body Airway Management

In the *Pediatric Airway Management Study*, a prehospital trial of airway management techniques in 830 infants and children, there were 22 (2.65%) enrolled patients who required airway management (bag-mask ventilation or endotracheal intubation) for foreign body aspiration. Types of foreign bodies encountered in this study included: superball (3), hotdog (3), marble (3), balloon (2), popcorn (2), grape (2), tooth (1), turkey meat (1), chicken meat (1), pasta (1), bolt (1), and licorice (1) (Figure 6-1). Other studies have shown that fatal foreign body aspiration is most often caused by balloons, balls, marbles, and other toys (Figure 6-2).

In the *Pediatric Airway Management Study*, patients with foreign body aspiration had a significantly improved neurological outcome if they were *not* intubated after the foreign body had been removed with Magill forceps. It is possible that attempts at intubation after the foreign body has been removed create further hypoxic stress on an already hypoxic heart and brain. BLS maneuvers were successful in removing two of the foreign bodies and ALS maneuvers were attempted 11 times and were successful in removing nine foreign bodies from the airway. This is why it is recommended to begin with BLS maneuvers first but then to quickly move to ALS procedures to remove the foreign body.

Recommendations and guidelines for the use of these BLS and ALS obstructed airway procedures and techniques are described in the 2000 American Heart Association Guidelines, *The Pediatric Airway Management Course*, the EMT-B Basic and Paramedic National Standard Curriculum, the Teaching Resource for Instructors in Prehospital Pediatrics (TRIPP), and the Pediatric Education for Prehospital Professionals (PEPP) Course Textbook and on-line renewal.

---

1. Gausche M, Lewis RJ, Stratton SJ, et al. Effect of out-of-hospital pediatric endotracheal intubation on survival and neurological outcome: A controlled clinical trial. *JAMA*. 2000;283:6:783–790.
2. Rimell FL, Thorne A, Stool S, et al. Characteristics of objects that cause choking in children. *JAMA*. 1995;274:1763–1766.

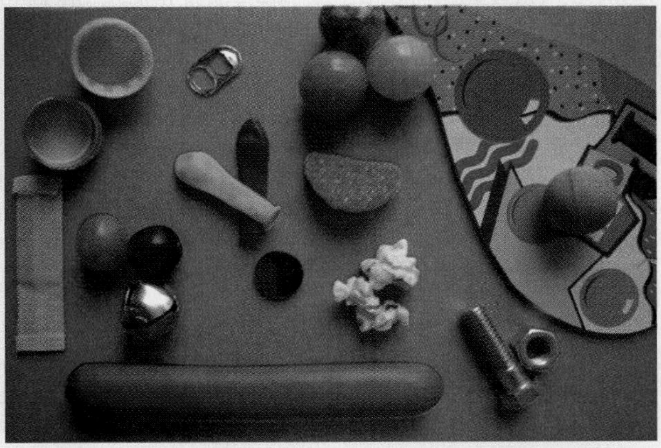

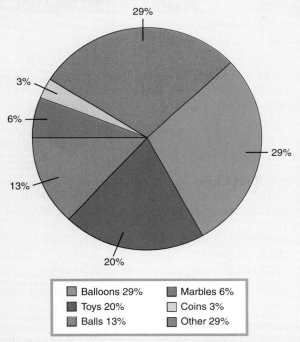

29%

3%

6%

29%

13%

20%

Balloons 29%   Marbles 6%
Toys 20%   Coins 3%
Balls 13%   Other 29%

Figure 6-2 Types of objects causing choking deaths in children.[2]

Figure 6-1 Examples of foreign bodies obstructing the airway in children.

- The larynx (glottis), located higher in the neck of infants and young children
- The cricoid ring, the narrowest portion of the airway
- The tracheal diameter that is smaller, and the tracheal rings that are more compressible
- The lower airways that are smaller in diameter

The narrowest portion of the pediatric airway is the cricoid ring located below the level of the vocal cords. The tracheal rings, which provide structure and strength in the adult airway, are more compressible and collapse easily in children. A large foreign body in the esophagus can therefore push against the trachea, compressing the airway and leading to airway obstruction (Figure 6-3). The lower airways are smaller in diameter and thus are more easily occluded. Combining these anatomic differences with the natural tendency for children (especially those under 3

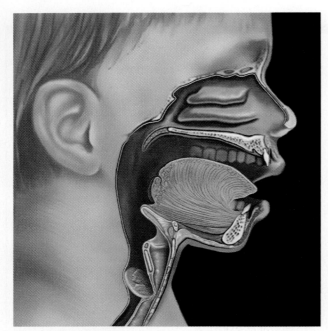

Figure 6-3 A large foreign body in the esophagus can press on a child's trachea, obstructing the airway.

years of age) to put objects in their mouths, it is easy to see why foreign body airway obstruction is not uncommon.

Indications

Conscious Child

Indications for BLS maneuvers to clear an upper airway foreign body obstruction in a conscious child include:

- Sudden onset of respiratory distress characterized by:
  - Coughing, gagging, and/or stridor with aphonia

Unconscious Child

Indications for BLS maneuvers to clear an upper airway foreign body obstruction in an unconscious child include:

- Inability to ventilate

Presence of a foreign body causing airway obstruction must be considered whenever the above finding is noted. It is possible for an object to obstruct the upper airway at any point from the back of the throat to the trachea. The object may be located within the airway itself or within the esophagus. For any foreign body resulting in complete upper airway obstruction, begin with BLS maneuvers to dislodge the foreign body from the level of obstruction to the oropharynx. If the object is lodged in the upper portion of the esophagus, it can push against the trachea, collapsing it and resulting in a partial or complete airway obstruction. In

this situation direct laryngoscopy will be ineffective because the object is not located within the airway and therefore cannot be visualized. Using BLS maneuvers, you may dislodge the object in the esophagus, allowing it to come back up into the oropharynx, where it may be removed. In the field setting this may be the only treatment option available.

Contraindications

Contraindications for BLS maneuvers to clear an upper airway foreign body obstruction include:

- Coughing, gagging, and/or stridor *with* the ability to speak, cry, or cough

Avoid any airway interventions in a child who still has the ability to speak, cry and/or cough, as you may end up converting a partial obstruction into a complete obstruction. Transport these patients immediately. Provide 100% oxygen as tolerated, avoiding any agitation of the child.

Procedure Step-by-Step

video This section discusses BLS procedures first, followed by ALS.

Complete Obstruction: Conscious Infant (0–1 yr)

Holding the infant securely, place the infant on your forearm, face down with your hand supporting the face/chin in a head-down position. With the opposite hand, deliver five back blows between the shoulder blades using the heel of your hand (Figure 6-4).

Sandwiching the infant between your two forearms, turn him on his back, supporting the occiput with your hand. Open the infant's mouth and remove the foreign body if it is visible. Do not perform blind finger sweeps, as this may result in pushing the foreign body further into the airway.

If no foreign body is visible, deliver five chest thrusts using your index and middle finger placed on the lower third of the sternum, at the nipple line to one fingerbreadth below (Figure 6-5).

Open the infant's mouth and remove the foreign body if it is visible. If no foreign body is visible, repeat cycles of back blows and chest thrusts until the foreign body is removed or the infant becomes unconscious.

The steps for managing complete obstruction in a conscious infant are summarized as follows:

1. Perform back blows.
2. Remove the visible foreign body.
3. Perform chest thrusts if no foreign body is visible.
4. Remove the visible foreign body.
5. Repeat back blows and chest thrusts until the foreign body is removed or the infant becomes unconscious.

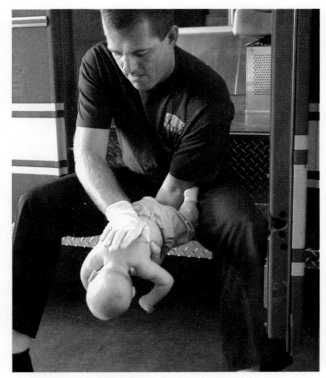

Figure 6-4 Perform back blows (infant).

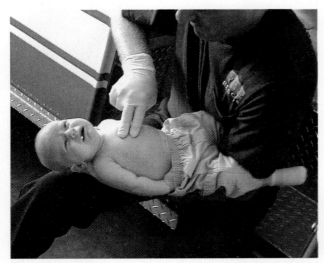

Figure 6-5 Perform chest thrusts if no foreign body is visible (infant).

Complete Obstruction: Unconscious Infant (0–1 yr)

Position the infant supine in a neutral sniffing position on a flat, firm surface. Open the mouth using thumb pressure on the chin.

Look into the mouth and remove the foreign object, if seen. Attempt to ventilate with a bag-mask device. If unsuccessful, reposition the infant and attempt to ventilate again. If still unsuccessful, begin cycles of back blows and chest thrusts.

Examine the oropharynx for a foreign body and if visualized, remove it. Continue cycles of back blows

and chest thrusts until the object is dislodged or until ALS foreign body airway obstruction removal procedures can be performed.

The steps for managing complete obstruction in an unconscious infant are summarized as follows:

1. Remove the visible foreign body.
2. Attempt to ventilate with bag-mask device.
3. Reposition.
4. Repeat attempt to ventilate.
5. Begin cycles of five back blows and five chest thrusts with attempts to ventilate between each.
6. Perform ALS procedures if the airway is still obstructed after at least one cycle of BLS maneuvers has failed to relieve the obstruction.

Complete Obstruction: Conscious Child

Stand behind the child and wrap your arms around the chest, below the axillae. Make a fist with one hand and place the thumb side of your fist against the child's abdomen, just above the navel. To prevent injury, avoid placing your hand near the xiphoid process. Using your other hand, grasp your fist and perform five abdominal thrusts in an upward direction. Continue to perform abdominal thrusts until the foreign body is dislodged or until the child loses consciousness.

The steps for managing complete obstruction in a conscious child are summarized as follows:

1. Stand behind the child.
2. Place your arms around the child's chest.
3. Place one fist with your thumb against the child's abdomen, below the xiphoid and above the navel.
4. Grasp your fist with your other hand.
5. Give five abdominal thrusts in an upward direction (Figure 6-6).

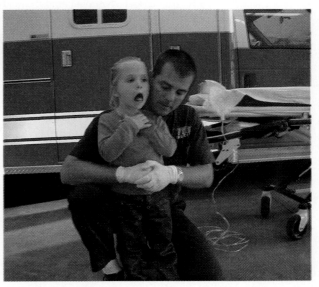

Figure 6-6 Give five abdominal thrusts in an upward direction (child).

6. Continue abdominal thrusts until the foreign body is dislodged or the child becomes unconscious.

Complete Obstruction: Unconscious Child

Place the child supine in neutral position on a firm, flat surface. Open the mouth using thumb pressure on the chin and look for a foreign body. If a foreign body is observed, remove it. Do not perform blind finger sweeps **(Figure 6-7)**.

Attempt to ventilate with a bag-mask device **(Figure 6-8)**. If there is no chest rise with ventilation, reposition and attempt ventilation again. If you are still unable to ventilate, kneel beside, or straddle, the child. Place the heel of your open hand above the navel just below the xiphoid process. Put your other hand on top of the first hand and interlock your fingers.

Give five quick upward abdominal thrusts, avoiding the xiphoid process **(Figure 6-9)**. Open the airway and look for a foreign body in the mouth. If a foreign body is observed, remove it **(Figure 6-10)**. Do not perform blind finger sweeps.

Attempt to ventilate. If unable to ventilate, repeat abdominal thrusts until object is dislodged or until ALS foreign body airway obstruction removal procedures can be performed.

The steps for managing complete obstruction in an unconscious child are summarized as follows:

1. Place the child supine.
2. Look for a foreign body; remove if seen.
3. Attempt to ventilate.
4. Reposition.
5. Repeat attempt to ventilate.
6. Kneel beside, or straddle, the child.
7. Place the heel of the open hand below the xiphoid and above the navel.
8. Place the second hand on top of the first, fingers interlaced.
9. Perform five quick upward abdominal thrusts.
10. Look for the foreign body and remove it. Do not perform blind finger sweeps.
11. Attempt to ventilate.

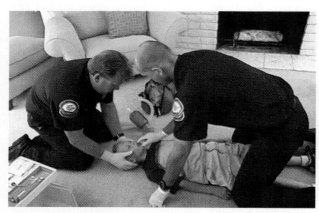

Figure 6-7 Begin BLS maneuvers to remove an airway foreign body in an unconscious child by placing the child supine in neutral position and opening the mouth using thumb pressure on the chin to look for a foreign body.

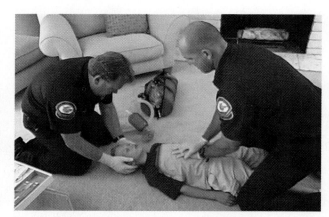

Figure 6-9 Perform five quick upward abdominal thrusts.

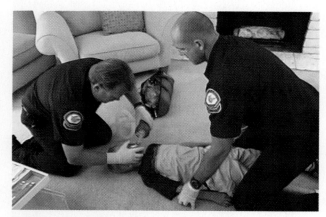

Figure 6-8 Attempt to ventilate.

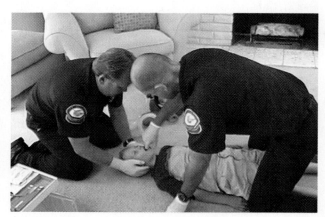

Figure 6-10 Look for the foreign body and remove it.

12. Continue abdominal thrusts until the foreign body is dislodged or you are ready to begin ALS procedures.

ALS Foreign Body Airway Obstruction Removal

Continue to attempt ventilation with a bag-mask device. Prepare the equipment. Select the pediatric laryngoscope handle and the appropriate size blade. Check the laryngoscope bulb to ensure that the light is functioning and is tightly screwed in to the handle ("bright and tight"). Select the pediatric, closed-tipped Magill forceps. Ensure that the suction equipment is operational.

Place the child supine on a firm, flat surface in a neutral sniffing position. Open the child's mouth by using your thumb to apply downward pressure to the chin. Insert the laryngoscope in the mouth. Hold the laryngoscope blade just to the left of the midline. This will create more room on the right side of the mouth for insertion of the Magill forceps.

Use a lifting motion, not a prying motion, with the laryngoscope blade to visualize the posterior pharynx and vocal cords. If the foreign body is not visible, suction the oropharynx to improve visibility while being careful not to push the foreign body deeper into the airway. Monitor the patient's heart rate. Bradycardia may occur due to hypoxia or manipulation of the posterior pharynx.

If a foreign body is visualized, remove it with the Magill forceps. Insert the pediatric Magill forceps with the tips closed into the right corner of the mouth. The tips must be closed to avoid causing injury during insertion. Observing the tips of the forceps at all times, open the Magill forceps around the foreign object and attempt to grasp the object. Grasp the object and carefully remove it from the mouth. Suction as needed. Be aware that as the object is removed, the potential for vomiting and aspiration is high.

After removal of the object, reposition the patient and attempt to ventilate with a bag-mask device. If you are able to ventilate the patient, check for a pulse. If a pulse is present, continue to assist ventilation and observe for signs of improvement, such as the return of spontaneous respiration. If no pulse is present, begin CPR. If you are unable to ventilate the patient, reposition, and attempt ventilation again. If still unable to ventilate, repeat ALS procedures using a laryngoscope and Magill forceps to remove all obstructing objects from the airway.

There may be multiple pieces or multiple objects that need to be removed. If the foreign object is located below the level of the vocal cords, do not attempt to remove it using the laryngoscope and Magill forceps, but attempt to dislodge it above the vocal cords using BLS maneuvers.

The steps for ALS foreign body airway removal are summarized as follows:

1. Gather the equipment: Laryngoscope and blade, Magill forceps, suction equipment.
2. Place the patient in a supine position.
3. Insert the laryngoscope in the right side of the mouth, sweep tongue to midline. Attempt to visualize the object. Insert the Magill forceps with the tips closed into the right side of the mouth.
4. Grasp and remove the foreign body.
5. Suction as needed.
6. Reassess.
7. Attempt to ventilate.
8. Repeat the procedure as needed until all foreign objects are removed and you are able to ventilate the patient.
9. Begin CPR as needed.

ALS foreign body airway management is summarized in **Skill Drill 6-1**.

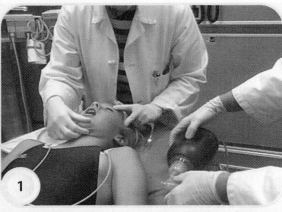

1 To begin ALS maneuvers to remove an airway foreign body, open the child's mouth by using your thumb to apply downward pressure to the chin.

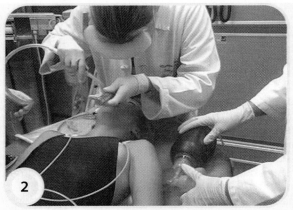

2 If the foreign body is not visible, suction the oropharynx to improve visibility while being careful not to push the foreign body deeper into the airway.

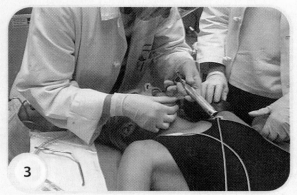

3 Insert the laryngoscope blade in the mouth to visualize the posterior pharynx and vocal cords or to visualize the foreign body in the airway.

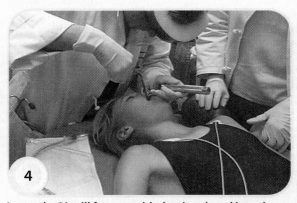

4 Insert the Magill forceps with the tips closed into the right side of the mouth.

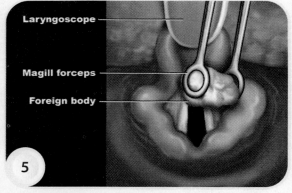

Laryngoscope

Magill forceps

Foreign body

5 Open the Magill forceps around the foreign object and attempt to grasp the object.

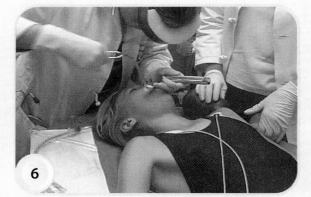

6 Grasp the object and carefully remove it from the mouth.

■ Problem Solving

Use the following approaches to resolve problems that may occur during foreign body removal:

- If you do not have enough room on the side of the patient's mouth to insert the Magill forceps, move the laryngoscope blade slightly to the left of the midline or ask your partner to retract, with his/her gloved small finger, the patient's cheek at the corner of the mouth.

- If you have difficulty visualizing the whole airway, lift the laryngoscope blade with the muscles of your upper arm, flexing at the elbow and moving the tongue and lower jaw upward. This movement allows for greater visualization of the airway. Do not flex the wrist—this will move the tip of the blade toward you, causing the tongue to fall backward into the airway.

- In some very rare circumstances if the object is below the vocal cords, some textbooks suggest pushing the object into the right mainstem bronchus with an endotracheal tube. This should NOT be attempted unless all BLS and ALS maneuvers have failed. *The problem with this desperate procedure is that the object may be pushed deep into the trachea so that even needle cricothyrotomy or tracheostomy will not relieve the obstruction. In this case, there would be irreversible airway obstruction and the patient would die.*

Complications

Possible complications resulting from foreign body airway removal include:
- Converting a partial obstruction to a complete obstruction
- Trauma to chest and abdomen
- Forcing the object deeper into the airway
- Trauma to the soft tissues of the airway and/or broken teeth

Converting a Partial Obstruction to a Complete Obstruction

As serious as a foreign body airway obstruction is, the procedures used to relieve it are not without potential for serious complications. Trying to intervene rather than providing supportive measures when the airway is only partially obstructed can convert a situation where there is some oxygenation and ventilation to complete airway obstruction where oxygenation and ventilation are not possible without removal of the foreign object.

Trauma to the Chest and Abdomen

Improper hand position during BLS maneuvers can fracture the rib(s), sternum, and/or xyphoid process, which can result in a pneumothorax or cardiac injury. Even if

there are no fractures, it is possible to cause injuries to abdominal organs such as the liver and spleen.

Forcing the Object Deeper into the Airway

A foreign object can be forced deeper into the airway by inappropriate interventions (Figure 6-11), such as by placing an oropharyngeal airway. Blind finger sweeps can force the object further down; an attempt to do this deliberately as a last ditch effort to push the object into the right mainstem bronchus also carries the risk of causing complete irreversible airway obstruction. The best way to prevent these complications is to use all airway interventions thoughtfully and appropriately; the goal is not to cause further injury.

Trauma to the Soft Tissues of the Airway and/or Broken Teeth

In order to prevent trauma to the soft tissues of the airway and/or broken teeth, give 100% oxygen as tolerated in cases of partial obstruction and do not attempt BLS or ALS maneuvers unless the patient's condition deteriorates. Do not perform blind finger sweeps, and use proper hand placement while performing all BLS maneuvers. Careful airway management can prevent injury and additional complications.

It can be difficult to resist the urge to use the laryngoscope and Magill forceps before BLS maneuvers have been performed. If you clearly understand the differences between pediatric and adult airway anatomy, however, and you remember that the foreign body may actually be in the esophagus, you should attempt BLS maneuvers once before beginning ALS maneuvers. Then quickly attempt ALS maneuvers and if the foreign body is not visualized in the airway to the vocal cords it may be below the cords or in the esophagus. It is critical to then attempt BLS maneuvers again, to dislodge the foreign body, and if you are not able to dislodge the object consider needle cricothyrotomy.

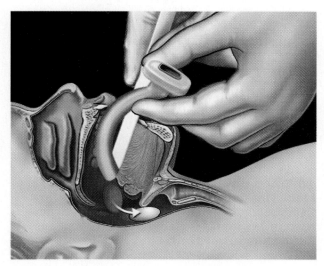

Figure 6-11 An object can be pushed further into the airway, creating a complete obstruction, if an inappropriate intervention is used.

Conclusions

Historically, training provided for prehospital providers has had difficulty recreating, with any sense of realism, the emotions, stress, and actual difficulties encountered in coping with pediatric airway obstruction. Removing a piece of sponge or other simulated foreign body from the airway of a pediatric manikin in a classroom setting will never adequately approximate the reality of working in a less than ideal environment while trying to remove a slippery object from a tiny airway. Practicing skills, however, may help to ensure that airway management will be performed correctly when needed.

You need to have a high index of suspicion for foreign body airway obstruction, and be able to perform airway management procedures in proper sequence, for the infant or child to have the best chance of a good outcome. Remember, when there is prolonged airway obstruction, even when you perform all procedures correctly and in a timely fashion, the outcome may be dismal.

Scenario Review

You have responded to a private residence and found law enforcement personnel performing CPR on a 4-year-old boy. Your initial assessment revealed that the boy was apneic but had a pulse rate of 80 beats per minute. CPR was discontinued. Attempts at ventilation with bag-mask device failed to cause the chest to rise even when the patient was repositioned.

1. *What are the possible reasons for a lack of chest rise?*

Airway obstruction, improper head and neck positioning, the need for an airway adjunct due to loss of muscle tone, and equipment failure can all lead to the inability to obtain adequate chest rise.

2. *What are your immediate interventions?*

Reposition the head and neck and attempt to ventilate again.

Consider the possibility that a foreign body airway obstruction exists. Because the child is apneic, you begin with one cycle of abdominal thrusts. You are unable to visualize an object in the mouth and you are still unable to ventilate. You instruct one of your team members to perform abdominal thrusts while you gather a pediatric laryngoscope, pediatric Magill forceps, and suction. When you place the laryngoscope in the mouth and attempt to visualize the airway, you notice a round object obstructing the child's airway. You remove the object, which turns out to be a superball, and attempt to ventilate once again. This time you note chest rise and normal resistance, and are able to auscultate breath sounds bilaterally with bag-mask ventilation. You reassess the heart rate, which increases from 60 to 140 beats per minute with bag-mask ventilation. You transport the child to the hospital; en route the child becomes more alert and pushes your hand away. You provide 100% oxygen by partial nonrebreather mask and the child sits up.

The paramedics did an excellent job of considering the possibility of a foreign body airway obstruction when they were unable to adequately ventilate the child.

This case provides two good teaching points:

1. If you cannot ventilate the patient, you must consider the possibility of an airway obstruction.
2. Begin with BLS maneuvers to dislodge a foreign body. If this intervention is unsuccessful, quickly move to ALS maneuvers to clear the foreign object from the airway.

Quick Quiz

1. *Which of the following are indicative of a complete foreign body airway obstruction?*
   - A. Gradual onset of symptoms
   - B. Equal breath sounds bilaterally
   - C. Inability to make any sound or to speak
   - D. Crying, coughing, and/or wheezing
   - E. Normal skin color

2. *Which one of the following is contraindicated when attempting to remove a foreign body airway obstruction?*
   - A. Insertion of the Magill forceps in the right side of the mouth.
   - B. Performing BLS procedures prior to attempting laryngoscopy.
   - C. Using Magill forceps to remove a foreign body visualized below the vocal cords.
   - D. Placing your hand(s) below a child's xiphoid process and above the navel when performing abdominal thrusts.
   - E. Supporting the infant's occiput with your hand when performing chest thrusts.

3. *Which of the following is not a potential complication of BLS foreign body airway obstruction procedures?*
   - A. Conversion of a partial obstruction to a complete obstruction
   - B. Rib, sternum, and/or xiphoid fracture
   - C. Pneumothorax
   - D. Aspiration of stomach contents
   - E. Bruising of the abdomen and chest

4. *After performing five back blows and opening the child's mouth, you may attempt a blind finger sweep in an attempt to locate the foreign body.*
   - A. True
   - B. False

Glossary

aphonia Voice loss.

auscultate To listen to sounds within the body, usually with a stethoscope.

axilla (plural = axillae) The armpit.

bradycardia A slow heartbeat.

laryngoscopy An examination of the interior of the larynx, usually done with a laryngoscope.

oropharynx The area of the pharynx located between the soft palate and upper part of the epiglottis.

xiphoid process The sword-shaped piece of cartilage located at the lower end of the sternum.

Selected References

1. American Heart Association. 2000 American Heart Association Guidelines, *Circulation.* 2000;102 (suppl I):I-253–I-290.

2. American Heart Association. American Heart Association guidelines for cardiopulmonary resuscitation and emergency cardiovascular care: Pediatric basic life support and pediatric advanced life support. *Circulation.* 2000;102(8);I-253–I-342.

3. Bank DE, Krug SE. New approaches to upper airway disease. *Emerg Med Clinics NA.* 1995;13:473–487.

4. Byard RW. Mechanisms of unexpected death in infants and young children following foreign body ingestion. *JFSCA.* 1996;41:438–441.

5. Committee on Pediatric Emergency Medicine. First aid for the choking child. *Pediatrics.* 1993;93:477–479.

6. Dieckmann RA, Brownstein D, Gausche-Hill M, eds. *Pediatric Education for Prehospital Professionals: PEPP Textbook.* Sudbury, Mass: Jones and Bartlett Publishers; 2000.

7. Foltin G, Tunik M, Cooper A, eds. *Teaching Resource for Instructors in Prehospital Pediatrics (EMT-Basic).* New York: Maternal and Child Health Bureau Center for Pediatric Emergency Medicine; 1998.

8. Gausche M, Goodrich SM, Poore PD, eds. *Instructor Manual for Advanced Life Support Providers: Pediatric Airway Management Project.* 2nd ed. Washington, D.C.: Maternal and Child Health Bureau, National Highway Traffic and Safety Administration, and the Agency for Healthcare Research and Quality; 1997.

9. Gausche M, Goodrich SM, Poore PD, eds. *Instructor Manual for Basic Life Support Providers: Pediatric Airway Management Project.* 1st ed. Washington, D.C.: Maternal and Child Health Bureau, National Highway Traffic and Safety Administration, and the Agency for Healthcare Research and Quality; 1997.

10. Gausche M, Lewis RJ, Stratton SJ, et al. Effect of out-of-hospital pediatric endotracheal intubation on survival and neurological outcome: A controlled clinical trial. *JAMA.* 2000;283:6:783–790.

11. Gausche-Hill M, Dieckmann RA, Brownstein D, eds. *Pediatric Education for Prehospital Professionals: PEPP Resource Manual.* Sudbury, Mass: Jones and Bartlett Publishers; 2000.

12. Rimell FL, Thorne A, Stool S, et al. Characteristics of objects that cause choking in children. *JAMA.* 1995;274:1763–1766.

13. Shirm SW. Emergency maneuvers for airway obstruction by foreign body. In: Dieckmann RA, Fiser DH, Selbst SM, eds. *Pediatric Emergency & Critical Care Procedures.* St. Louis, Mo: Mosby-Year Book, Inc.; 1997.

14. Todres DI, Pediatric airway control and ventilation. *Ann Emerg Med.* 1993;22:440–444.

15. Weiss RL, Goldstein MN, Dharia A, et al. Clear plastic cups: A childhood choking hazard. *Int J of Pediatr Otorhinolaryngol* 1996;37:243–251.

16. Yeh TS, Andropoulos DB. Upper airway obstruction. In: Dieckmann RA, Fiser DH, Selbst SM, eds. *Pediatric Emergency & Critical Care Procedures.* St. Louis: Mosby-Year Book, Inc.; 1997.

End of Chapter Activities

Technology Resources

Online Course

Anatomy Review

Online Glossary

Web Links

Online Quiz

Scenarios

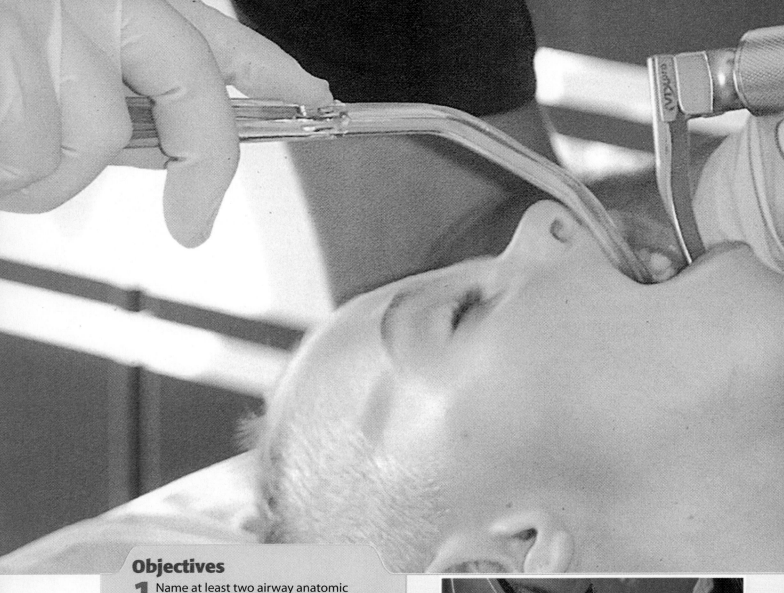

Objectives

1 Name at least two airway anatomic differences between adults and children that may affect your approach to endotracheal intubation.

2 Name two actions necessary in preparing to intubate the pediatric patient.

3 Describe the selection of the appropriate size of endotracheal tube.

4 Identify two complications of endotracheal intubation.

5 Discuss the indications and contraindications of endotracheal intubation.

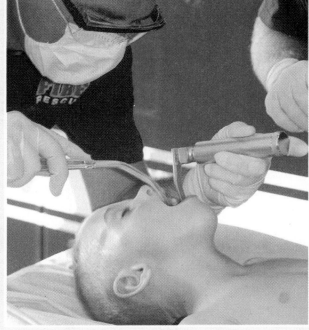

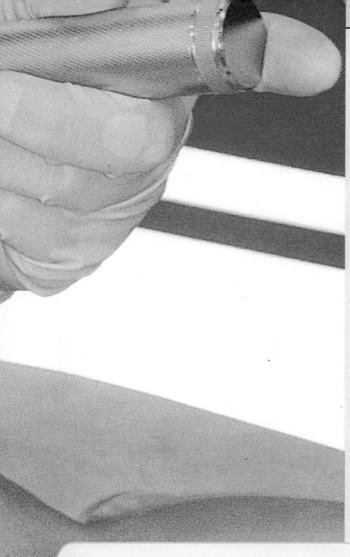

CHAPTER 7

Endotracheal Intubation

Scenario

You are called to the home of an 11-month-old girl. Upon arrival, the mother leads you to the child's bedroom where you find her cyanotic with very little chest movement. There is vomitus containing white powdery fragments on the carpet. The mother tells you the child may have swallowed some sleeping pills. You position the child's head to open the airway, and suction vomitus from the airway. She has a strong pulse. Despite bag-mask ventilation, oxygen saturation shown on the pulse oximeter remains at 85%. Your protocols include endotracheal intubation as an option for management of respiratory failure.

1. *What initial actions would you take to manage this child's airway?*

2. *How would you determine that your airway management is effective?*

Think about these questions and this case as you read on. We will return to this scenario at the end of the chapter.

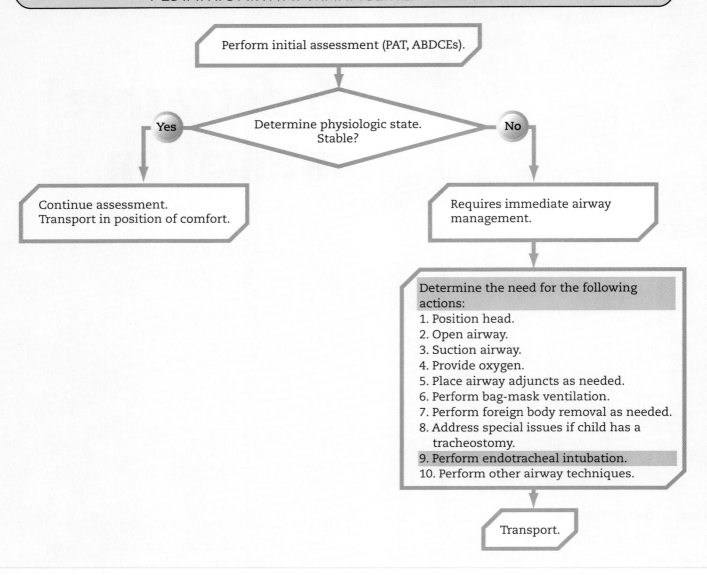

Perform initial assessment (PAT, ABDCEs).

Determine physiologic state. Stable?

Yes

No

Continue assessment.
Transport in position of comfort.

Requires immediate airway management.

Determine the need for the following actions:
1. Position head.
2. Open airway.
3. Suction airway.
4. Provide oxygen.
5. Place airway adjuncts as needed.
6. Perform bag-mask ventilation.
7. Perform foreign body removal as needed.
8. Address special issues if child has a tracheostomy.
9. Perform endotracheal intubation.
10. Perform other airway techniques.

Transport.

Introduction

While many children need immediate airway management, few will require immediate endotracheal intubation. Endotracheal intubation should always be preceded by other less invasive attempts at airway management, particularly the use of bag-mask ventilation. Because of the risks of endotracheal intubation, such as esophageal intubation and damage to the airway, its use should be carefully considered and balanced against the risks involved and the prolongation of scene time.

Anatomical Considerations

video Anatomical differences between the adult and pediatric patient impact the approach and equipment choices during endotracheal intubation. Here are some important differences between the adult and pediatric airways:

- The prominent occiput of the infant or child will often necessitate elevating the shoulders to align the airway axes. Appropriate alignment facilitates intubation.
- Tracheal rings are elastic and collapse more easily in children versus adults. Hyperextension of the head may actually cause airway compromise as the tracheal rings collapse. Appropriate positioning of the head may relieve airway obstruction and make endotracheal intubation unnecessary.
- The tongue of the infant or child is larger in proportion to the mouth. Improper positioning of

Problems with Endotracheal Intubation

Although bag-mask ventilation and endotracheal intubation are widely used in the prehospital setting, there are only a few studies that have evaluated the efficacy of these procedures systematically. However, some important facts do emerge from a review of these studies:

- Success rates for pediatric endotracheal intubation vary greatly (50% to 95%). Most studies report that success rates are lower with younger ages, specifically at younger than one year of age.
- Complication rates reported vary from 2% to 25%. Dislodgement of the endotracheal tube into the mouth, posterior pharynx, or esophagus may occur in as many as 15% of patients. While the use of end-tidal CO_2 detectors may help reduce these complications, studies show that despite their use, the complication is not completely eliminated.
- Paramedics trained in intubation will apply the skill only 70% of the time that patients meet indications for the procedure. So, even when the skill is available, pediatric patients are often managed with basic airway management.
- Prolongation in scene times with the use of endotracheal intubation varied from an added 2 minutes to over 10 minutes when compared with basic airway management.

- Intubation of pediatric trauma patients shows particularly high complication rates. Gastric distention occurs more frequently with bag-mask ventilation, yet the rates of vomiting or aspiration are comparable.
- Many pediatric patients who were intubated in the field may not have needed this procedure. In a review of the intubation of 605 pediatric trauma patients, Nakayama et al. reported that as many as 30% of the patients intubated had Glasgow Coma Scale scores of 10 or above with no apnea or airway compromise, suggesting that this procedure was unnecessary. Patients with seizures are the most likely to be extubated in the emergency department after field intubation. These children may have transient respiratory depression during the postictal state and may have needed only basic airway management such as positioning of the head, placement of a nasopharyngeal airway, and bag-mask ventilation.
- The largest prospective randomized trial comparing pediatric prehospital endotracheal intubation with bag-mask ventilation in an urban system did not show any improvement in survival or neurological outcome with the addition of endotracheal intubation to the paramedic scope of practice. In fact, there was improved survival when bag-mask ventilation alone was used for patients with respiratory arrest.

---

the laryngoscope blade can result in the tongue hiding the vocal cords.

- The epiglottis of the infant or child is floppy and protrudes into the pharynx. Using a curved laryngoscope blade for a child younger than 5 years of age may be more difficult because the epiglottis is not easily moved with elevation of the vallecula. A straight blade (Miller) may be the better choice in children.
- The smallest diameter of the airway in the pediatric patient is at the cricoid ring. For this reason, cuffed endotracheal tubes are generally not necessary for children younger than 8 years of age. The proper tube size will fit snugly at the level of the cricoid cartilage just below the vocal cords forming a seal without a cuff. Often there

is a small air leak. If the air leak is significant, then the endotracheal tube can be replaced in the emergency department with a half-sized larger tube.

Indications

The decision to intubate a patient should be based on careful clinical assessment. The most common indications for intubation may include:

- Respiratory arrest or failure not responding to bag-mask ventilation
- Cardiopulmonary arrest
- Head trauma patients requiring neurologic resuscitation (Glasgow Coma Scale score ≤ 9)

Contraindications

Contraindications to endotracheal intubation include:
- Permanent tracheostomy
- Adequate ventilation after basic airway interventions

Pre-intubation Procedures

The approach to management of any patient in respiratory distress or failure should be logical and sequential, beginning with basic airway maneuvers such as positioning, suctioning, and bag-mask ventilation. You may find, using this stepwise approach, that your patient requires **only** these maneuvers. Opening the airway may correct the underlying cause of airway distress, and more complex and invasive airway procedures may be unnecessary. When you decide that intubation is necessary, use the following steps.

Equipment

Ensure that the basic equipment is available while supporting respirations **(Table 7-1)**.

Choose the appropriate sized tube and laryngoscope blade using the length-based resuscitation tape, if available, or the following guidelines **(Figure 7-1)**. Either a curved or a straight blade may be used, but it is useful to have one size smaller and one size larger available **(Figure 7-2)**. Some general guidelines are:

- For term newborns, use a 3.0 or 3.5 mm tube.
- For an infant younger than six months of age use a 3.5 mm tube.
- By one year of age, a 4 mm tube can be used.
- The width of the small fingernail can be used to estimate the inside diameter of the tube **(Figure 7-3)**.
- Over one year of age the internal diameter of the tube can be estimated by the formula $(Age/4) + 4$.

A stylet may be used to stiffen the endotracheal tube during intubation. When used, insert the stylet

Table 7-1: Equipment for Endotracheal Intubation
Length-based resuscitation tape
Suction equipment
Suction tubing and tips
Laryngoscope and blades
Stylet
Pediatric Magill forceps
Endotracheal tubes (one size larger and smaller than indicated on length-based resuscitation tape)
Stethoscope
CO_2 detector, end-tidal CO_2 monitor and/or esophageal detector device
Oral airway
Cloth tape or commercially available endotracheal tube holder

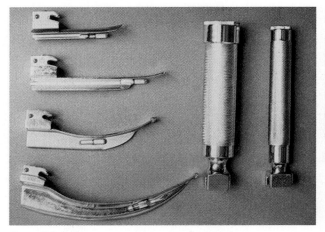

Figure 7-2 Curved and straight laryngoscope blades.

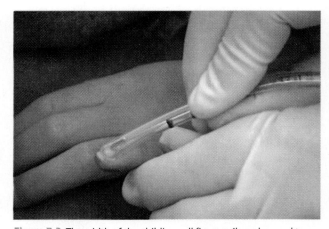

Figure 7-3 The width of the child's small fingernail can be used to estimate the inside diameter of the tube.

Figure 7-1 Close-up of the Broselow™ Pediatric Emergency Tape showing equipment appropriate for a child weighing between 12–14 kg.

to within 1 cm of the end of the tube and stabilize it by bending the end of the stylet against the upper lip of the endotracheal tube. Make sure the end of the stylet does not extend beyond the end of the tube. Otherwise, it could damage the airway structures.

Bend the endotracheal tube into a gentle curve, or bend the tip of the tube so that when it is inserted the tube goes more anterior toward the glottic opening (Figure 7-4). Ensure that suction is immediately available and that the device is working. Prepare the laryngoscope by attaching the blade to the handle and checking light operation. Make sure that pediatric Magill forceps are functioning and available. For a tube size 6.0 mm or greater, inflate the cuff with 10 mL of air, remove the syringe, feel for integrity of the balloon, reinsert the syringe, and deflate the balloon. Leave the syringe attached to the tube. Lubricate the tube with water-soluble lubricant.

Procedure Step-by-Step

video The steps for endotracheal intubation are described below and in **Skill Drill 7-1**.

The first step in endotracheal intubation is to apply cricoid pressure (Sellick maneuver) (Figure 7-5). This helps keep air from entering the stomach during bag-mask ventilation. Gentle pressure to the anterior neck (in a posterior direction) at the level of the cricoid cartilage closes off the esophagus and prevents air from entering. Preventing gastric distention aids ventilation by allowing maximum diaphragmatic excursion. It may also prevent passive movement of gastric contents up the esophagus and into the unprotected airway. The Sellick maneuver can be initiated along with bag-mask ventilation, and can continue through the intubation procedure. In some cases, the Sellick maneuver may also assist in visualization of the vocal cords by moving the cords posteriorly and upward during intubation. In infants, be careful not to apply excess pressure to the cricoid ring as excess pressure can collapse the cricoid ring and cause airway obstruction.

Position the child's head in a neutral position with in-line stabilization if you suspect head or neck trauma.

If no trauma is suspected, the patient can be placed in the sniffing position.

Instruct another provider to time the intubation attempts by giving 20 and 30 second counts (20 seconds to see the cords, plus 10 seconds to insert the tube). Open the child's mouth using thumb pressure on the chin. Place the laryngoscope in the right side of the patient's mouth and sweep the blade just to the left of the middle of the patient's upper lip (Figure 7-6).

Lift the patient's jaw with your laryngoscope without flexing your wrist, and visualize the airway. The blade may have to be advanced or withdrawn slightly in order to visualize the cords. Avoid using the upper teeth or gums as a fulcrum.

Advance the blade straight along the tongue until the tip is just beyond the epiglottis. If you are unable to visualize the vocal cords, ask another provider to retract the right corner of the patient's mouth with his or her small finger to assist in visualization. Once you visualize the cords, advance the tube through the cords.

Continue to advance the tube until the tube is just beyond the vocal cords (Figure 7-7). Avoid advancing the tube so far that it enters the <u>mainstem bronchus</u>:

- There are often cm markings on the side of the endotracheal tube for assessment of depth of tube placement (Figure 7-8).
- Correct depth of tube placement can be estimated from the length-based resuscitation tape or by using the formula CORRECT DEPTH = 3 times endotracheal tube size. For example, for a 1-year-old in which a 4.0 mm tube is placed, the estimated depth of tracheal tube placement is 12 cm. Always confirm proper depth and placement with clinical assessment followed by use of confirmation devices such as end-tidal or colorimetric CO_2 detectors.

Stabilize the tube against the upper lip, remove the stylet, and inflate the cuff (if the tube is over size 6.0 mm) (Figure 7-9). Confirm placement of the endotracheal tube using clinical assessment:

- Look for symmetrical chest rise.
- Listen for bubbling, gurgling sounds in the <u>epigastrium</u> for two breaths.

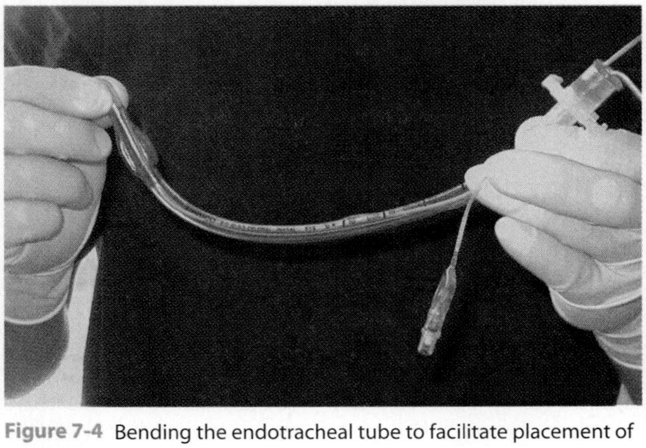

Figure 7-4 Bending the endotracheal tube to facilitate placement of the tube in the glottic opening.

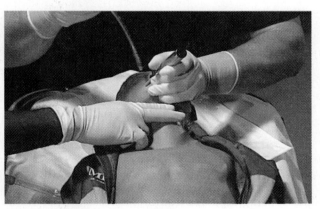
Figure 7-5 Applying cricoid pressure.

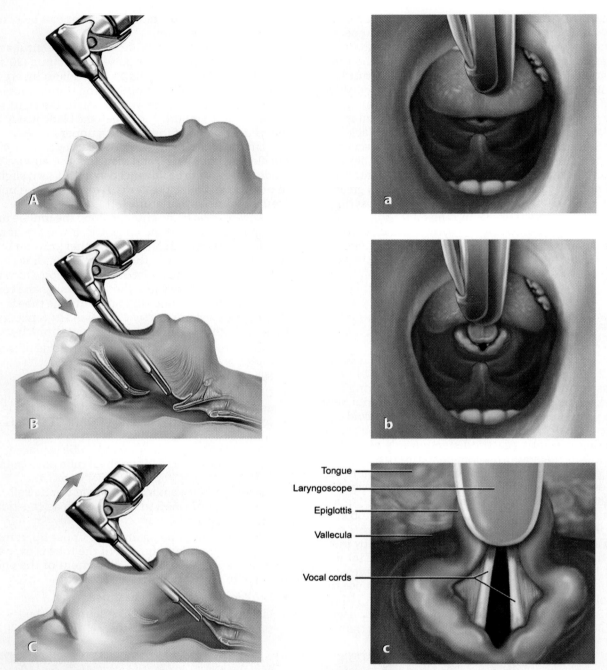

Figure 7-6 (A) Placing the laryngoscope blade. (B) View of the airway with the blade in the vallecula. (C) Continue to advance the laryngoscope blade until the epiglottis is lifted directly out of the visual plane of the airway and the cords are visualized. Two different views are shown for each of the three steps.

- Auscultate the chest in the third intercostal space, mid-axillary line for at least two breaths on each side.

Confirm placement with colorimetric end-tidal CO_2 device, end-tidal CO_2 monitoring, or use of an esophageal detector device (Figure 7-10). Once the tube has been confirmed to be in the trachea, secure it in place using tape or a commercially available endotracheal tube holder.

Confirmation of Endotracheal Tube Placement

Unrecognized dislodgment after placement has been reported to occur in as many as 6% of pediatric intubations, and esophageal intubation has been reported in 2% to 17% of cases, thus careful, systematic assessment of placement is essential. The most important confirmation of placement is visualization of the tube passing through the vocal cords. Immediately after

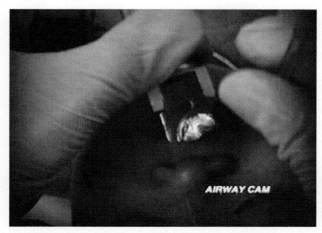

Figure 7-7 Advance the tube until the tube is just beyond the vocal cords.

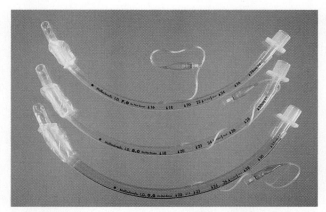

Figure 7-8 Size and cm markings are printed on the side of an endotracheal tube.

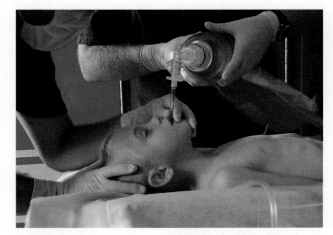

Figure 7-9 Stabilizing the endotracheal tube before taping.

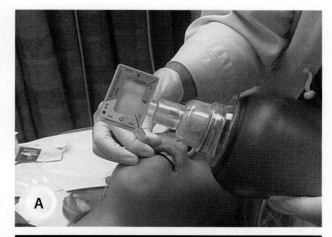

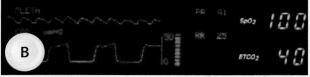

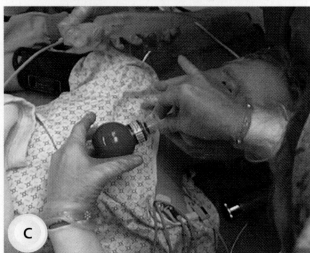

Figure 7-10 (A) Colorimetric end-tidal CO_2 detector. (B) End-tidal CO_2 device. (C) Esophageal detector bulb.

intubation, symmetrical chest rise and fall should also be observed. Listen to the stomach. If esophageal placement has occurred, you can hear gurgling sounds on insufflation when listening to the stomach — this is similar to the sound you hear when blowing through a drink-

ing straw into a glass of liquid. The gurgling sound may not be heard if the stomach is distended with air, so listen to the stomach before you listen to the lungs. If you hear breath sounds in the stomach, do not pull the tube as breath sounds are widely transmitted throughout the chest and abdomen even if the endotracheal tube is in the correct position. Only remove the endotracheal tube if gurgling sounds are heard. Continue your assessment. For lung auscultation, place your stethoscope over the second to third intercostal space, mid-axillary line on each side of the patient, and listen for breath sounds. Continue to auscultate the entire chest, listening for equal breath sounds bilaterally. There are additional methods for confirmation of tube placement.

Use of a Colorimetric CO_2 Detector Device

Colorimetric CO_2 detectors have been shown to be reliable in a non-cardiac arrest state, and can be used in an infant weighing as little as 2 kg. Adult detectors can be used to confirm placement, but should not be left in line for monitoring. The colorimetric CO_2 detector works by sensing when CO_2 passes through a special paper filter. The color of the paper changes from a baseline purple to yellow when CO_2 comes in contact with it (exhalation or release of the bag) and will return to purple when oxygen flows past it (inhalation or squeeze of the bag). With correct placement of the endotracheal tube, the CO_2 detector should turn yellow with exhalation and purple when 100% oxygen passes across the filter paper. As the patient is ventilated the detector will be purple then yellow, purple then yellow, and so on. Carbonated sodas have a high CO_2 content, which can result in initial detection of CO_2 values of greater than 2%, or tan on the colorimetric device. By the delivery of 6 additional breaths this retained CO_2 will be washed out and a more accurate reading can be made. If the reading is purple, suspect esophageal intubation; if tan, suspect a poor perfusion state, but with the tube in the trachea; if yellow, the tube is in the trachea.

The procedure for use of this device is as follows:

1. Determine correct size of CO_2 detector to be used.
   - Use a pediatric size detector for infants and children who weigh less than or equal to 15 kg (Figure 7-11); for children who weigh more than 15 kg, use the adult size

(Figure 7-12). Adult detectors can be used in infants as small as 2 kg to check endotracheal tube placement but cannot be left in-line as the device has a large amount of dead space (38 mL) that could lead to hypoventilation in the small infant. The pediatric detector has a small amount of dead space and is less bulky.

2. Attach the device to the upper end of the ETT and the other end to the bag-valve device.
3. Begin ventilation and clinical assessment.
4. Observe the CO_2 detector for color change during exhalation after 6 breaths have been delivered (Figure 7-13). Remember that the color will return to purple as you squeeze the bag and oxygen flows through the detector.
5. Your assessment of color change will determine the need for further intervention (Table 7-2).

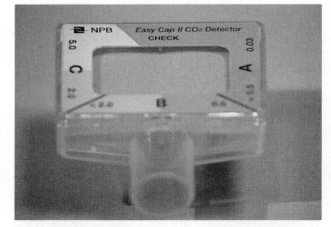

Figure 7-12 The adult CO_2 detector can be used in all children to confirm tracheal placement of the tube, but must be removed after 6 breaths in children with less than 15 kg body weight.

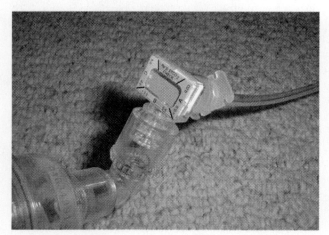

Figure 7-11 Pediatric CO_2 detector is used in infants and children weighing less than 15 kg.

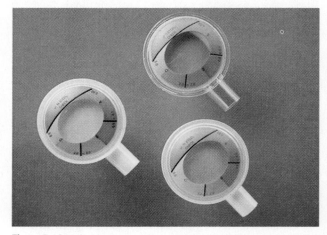

Figure 7-13 Color change on CO_2 detector with exhalation can assist the prehospital professional in determining the location of endotracheal tube.

Table 7-2: CO_2 Detection by Colors		
Color Change	Patient With a Pulse	Patient Without a Pulse
YELLOW	YES. The tube is in the trachea—leave in place and secure.	YES. The tube is in the trachea – leave in place and secure.
TAN	THINK. Think about possible causes of poor perfusion or poor CO_2 production as you deliver 6 more breaths. Also 6 breaths will wash out retained CO_2 in the stomach. If the color changes to yellow or remains tan, then YES, it is in the trachea. If color changes to purple, follow procedures for purple color change.	THINK. Think about possible causes of poor perfusion or poor CO_2 production as you deliver 6 more breaths. Also 6 breaths will wash out retained CO_2 in the stomach. If the color changes to yellow or remains tan, then YES, it is in the trachea. If color changes to purple, follow procedures for purple color change.
PURPLE	PROBLEM. The detector is not sensing CO_2, so the tube is in the esophagus; remove it.	PROBLEM. The detector is not sensing CO_2; causes may include misplacement of tube in the esophagus or the patient is not making any CO_2 as may occur in an arrest state. Revisualize the tube, if it is in the esophagus, remove it; if it is in the trachea, continue CPR.

Esophageal Detector Device

An aspiration bulb is used to apply suction to the end of the endotracheal tube to determine tracheal placement. The esophageal detector device can be a syringe or a bulb. With the syringe, as the syringe is pulled back, negative pressure is created which will collapse the esophagus causing resistance to pulling the syringe and thereby detecting esophageal placement. Because the adult trachea is held open by cartilage, negative pressure applied should result in free aspiration of air (Figure 7-14).

The self-inflating bulb works by the same principle. The bulb is compressed and then placed on the end of the endotracheal tube. If the tube is in the esophagus, the bulb will begin to fill but then stop, or fill very slowly as the walls of the esophagus collapse together with the application of negative pressure. If the tube is in the trachea the esophageal detector bulb should fill freely within 3 to 5 seconds (Figure 7-15).

The esophageal detector devices have been used in infants and children but because the tracheal walls in children collapse more easily and there is reduced exhaled volume of air, the bulb or syringe may not fill quickly, leading to a false conclusion that the tube is in the esophagus. These devices have been shown to be quite accurate in detecting tracheal or esophageal placement of the endotracheal tube in adults, but this method has not been adequately tested in children under 20 kg or 5 years of age.

When an esophageal detector device bulb or syringe is used, attach it to the end of the ETT if the child is greater than or equal to 20 kg bodyweight or 5 years of age; aspirate slowly over 3 to 5 seconds. If resistance is felt, then the tube is in the esophagus and should be removed; if air is aspirated, the ETT is in the trachea — secure the tube. This method, unlike with colorimetric devices, does not rely on physiologic production of CO_2 to determine tracheal placement of the endotracheal tube and is reliable in patients with cardiac arrest.

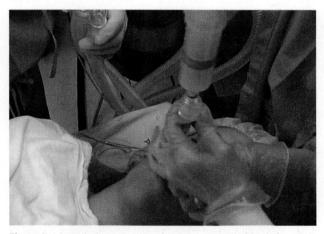

Figure 7-14 With the syringe, as the syringe is pulled back, free aspiration of air should occur if the endotracheal tube is in the trachea.

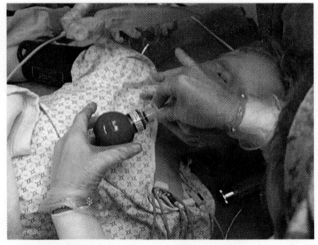

Figure 7-15 If the endotracheal tube is in the trachea, the esophageal detector bulb should fill freely within 3 to 5 seconds.

Use of Continuous End-tidal CO₂ Monitoring

This requires a special machine (capnometer) that continuously assesses the level of CO_2 at the end of the patient's exhalation. The capnometer uses an airway connector placed in-line with the patient's breathing circuit directly attached to the endotracheal tube. This technique produces instantaneous and accurate gas analysis. The normal values are 5% to 6% CO_2, which is equivalent to 35–45 mm Hg (Figure 7-16). A major advantage of this type of monitoring is that it can assist (along with clinical assessment) in determining not only whether the tube is in the trachea, but whether the patient's condition is improving or deteriorating over time.

Securing the Tube

Successful airway management requires correct securing of the tube after successful intubation. Securing the tube can be done by either taping or using a commercially available endotracheal tube holder (Figure 7-17). To secure the endotracheal tube with tape, one person should be assigned to hold the airway in place while the other tapes the tube. Place an oropharyngeal airway in patients who may bite the tube. Slide a long piece of cloth tape underneath the patient's neck, bring the first half of the tape up the side of the face close to the patient's mouth, and wrap it twice around the tube. Then bring the tape up the opposite side, cover a corner of the oropharyngeal airway (if used) as the tape comes across the upper lip, and wrap the tape twice around the tube. Fold over the ends of the tape to facilitate removal of the tape if the tube needs to be repositioned (Figure 7-18).

Reassess tube placement.

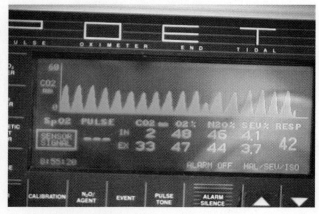

Figure 7-16 End-tidal CO_2 monitor showing exhaled CO_2 values in the normal range. Note that the inhaled value (upper number) is low because the patient is breathing gas mixed with high concentrations of oxygen.

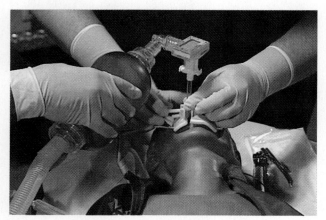

Figure 7-17 Endotracheal tube holders can be used to secure the tube in place.

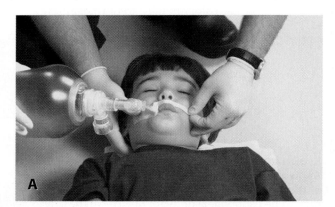

A

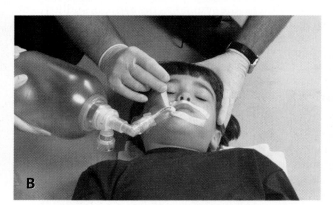

B

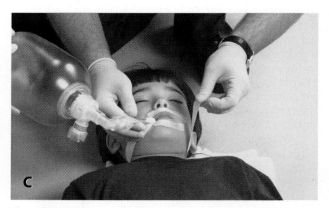

C

Figure 7-18 Taping technique for securing the endotracheal tube. Slide a long piece of cloth tape underneath the patient's neck. (A) Bring the first half of the tape up the side of the face close to the patient's mouth and wrap it twice around the tube. (B) Bring the tape up the opposite side and wrap the tape twice around the tube. (C) Reinforce the tape around the child's neck.

Preparation

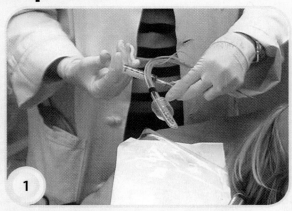

Assemble all equipment.

Select the appropriate size ET tube using tape, chart, or anatomic measurement.

Check the cuff for leaks (if less than 6.0 tube is used, do not test or inflate).

Inflate the cuff with 10 mL of air. Remove the syringe.

Feel the cuff for integrity while maintaining sterility. Deflate the cuff. Leave the syringe with 10 mL of air attached to the tube.

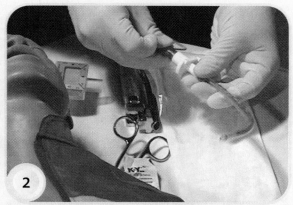

Recess the stylet at least 1 cm from the end of the tube and bend the tube into a gentle curve. Lubricate the tube with a water-soluble lubricant.

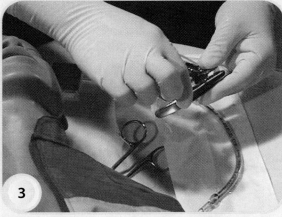

Attach the blade to the laryngoscope handle and ensure that the light is working.

Ensure that the suction device is functioning.

Instruct another provider to prepare for:

- Time counts (20 seconds to see cords, 30 seconds to insert ET tube)
- Handing the suction and ET tube
- Applying cricoid pressure
- Attaching the appropriate size CO_2 detector to manual resuscitator

Procedure

Complete Steps 4–7 in 20 seconds.

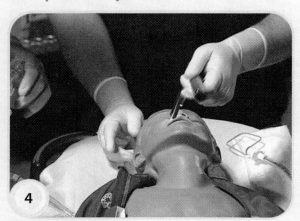

Position the patient:

Grasp the laryngoscope in your left hand.

Direct another provider to begin timing.

Open the patient's mouth using thumb pressure on the chin.

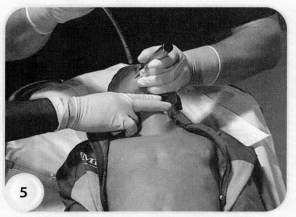

Ask another provider to apply cricoid pressure or apply it yourself.

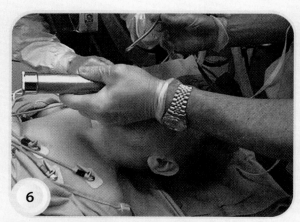

Insert a straight blade into the mouth, sweep the blade to the midline, and exert gentle traction upward.

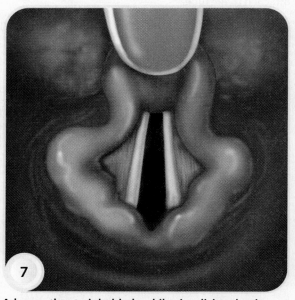

Advance the straight blade while visualizing the tip along the tongue until the tip is just beyond the epiglottis (epiglottis should not be visible if straight blade is correctly inserted).

Visualize the vocal cords; suction as needed.

Procedure—cont'd

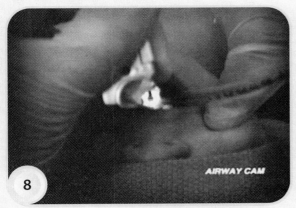

8

Carefully insert the tube in a dart-like fashion and advance the tube just beyond the cords.

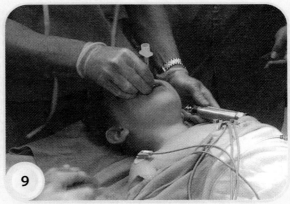

9

Remove the laryngoscope blade, carefully keeping the tube in place.

Remove the stylet, stabilizing the tube against the upper lip, being sure to secure the tube to the upper lip with your fingers. Never release the tube until it has been secured with tape or another stabilizing device.

Inflate cuff with pilot balloon, if using cuffed tube.

Confirmation of Tube Placement

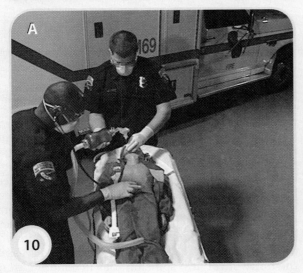

A

10

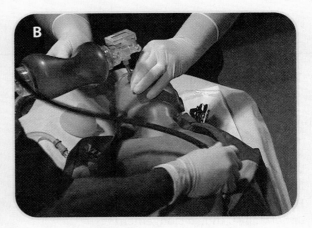

B

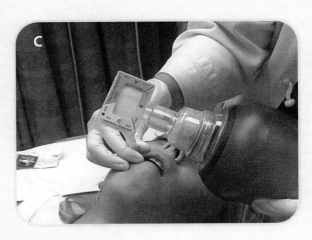

C

Place the CO_2 detector between the ET tube and the bag device.

Instruct another provider to ventilate with a bag device.

Observe for chest rise and fall.

Instruct another provider to maintain tube position and ventilate the patient.

Check tube placement by auscultating/observing for:

- Absence of gurgling noise in the epigastric area **(A)**
- Lung sounds bilaterally (3 ICS, mid-axillary line) **(B)**
- Observe the CO_2 detector color or capnography reading after a total of six breaths are delivered. **(C)**

Confirmation of Tube Placement—cont'd

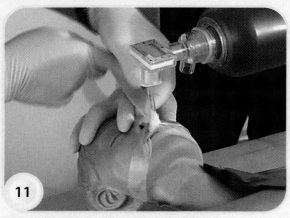

11

Initiate corrective measures as needed.

Note and record the tube position and CO_2 color detection.

Secure the ET tube with tape or an ET tube holder.

Reconfirm tube placement.

Remove the CO_2 detector if an adult detector is utilized. An appropriate size detector may be left in place.

■ Complications

Complications of endotracheal intubation include:
- Esophageal intubation
- Mainstem bronchus intubation
- Vomiting and aspiration
- Incorrect endotracheal tube size determination
- Hypoxia
- Endotracheal tube dislodgement
- Trauma to the mouth or airway structures

Proper training, skill maintenance, and experienced judgment all contribute to minimizing risks of this procedure. Gausche et al. demonstrated that in patients with respiratory arrest, survival rates with the use of bag-mask ventilation were better than with endotracheal intubation when there were short transport times. The frequency of vomiting (14%) and aspiration (15%) occurring during intubation are similar to that with bag-mask ventilation, while other complications, such as unrecognized esophageal intubation (2%), incorrect tube size (24%), and bronchial intubation (18%), are unique to endotracheal tube placement. Incorrect tube sizing can lead to a significant air leak around the tube and hypoventilation if the tube is too small, and injury to the airway if the tube is too large. In the younger age groups (younger than 18 months) there is a lower rate of successful intubation, often as low as 50%.

Endotracheal intubation involves the forceful manipulation of the upper airway with invasive instrumentation. Trauma to the teeth or gums can result from improper use of the laryngoscope. Mucosal surfaces bleed easily, and accidental lacerations or abrasions can cause obstruction or significant bleeding. Pneumothorax secondary to positive pressure ventilation can occur with bag-mask ventilation as well as with patients who are intubated and too aggressively ventilated. Despite the rarity of cervical spine injuries in children, worsening of an injury is always a consideration in trauma victims requiring airway management. The proper technique remains controversial; skilled intubation with in-line stabilization is considered to be an acceptable approach in patients with potential c-spine injury.

Endotracheal intubation should always be approached with the goal of preventing complications. Every intubation has the potential for complications, and the decision to perform this procedure requires balancing the inherent risks against the potential benefits to the patient. Once the critical decision has been made to perform the procedure, meticulous attention to proper equipment preparation and sizing (check and recheck), proper suction, length-based resuscitation tape guiding both tube selection and medication administration, cricoid pressure, pre-oxygenation, clinical assessment, and proper application of detector devices (CO_2 detector or esophageal bulb/syringe) will minimize complications. Timed attempts by an assistant can prevent prolonged attempts that can cause unintended hypoxia. Proper ventilation volume can minimize barotrauma (injury as a result of increased air pressure). Tube placement should be carefully confirmed (see confirmation of tube placement above).

Extubation should be performed if:

- There is no chest rise when ventilated.
- Bubbling, gurgling sounds are heard over the stomach.
- Breath sounds are absent bilaterally.
- CO_2 detector remains purple on exhalation in a patient with pulses or capnography values of less than 2%.

There is always the possibility that a patient may respond positively to resuscitation and require extubation. While not common, post-resuscitation extubation can be performed. Have suction ready for patients who demonstrate spontaneous respirations with adequate rate and tidal volume, regain consciousness, and begin to cough and gag.

Extubation

The first step in preparing to extubate is to ensure that the device is operating. Once this is done, the procedure for extubation occurs as follows:

- Suction the oropharynx.
- Turn the patient onto the left side.
- Deflate the cuff completely (if using a cuffed tube).
- Withdraw the tube rapidly at the end inspiratory phase while suctioning.

- Assess respiratory status.
- Continue to ventilate with a bag-mask device and consider re-intubation.

Endotracheal Drug Delivery

The use of the endotracheal tube for administration of medications has been a valuable alternative when there is a delay in intravenous access (Figure 7-19). Lidocaine, epinephrine, atropine, and naloxone (LEAN) can be administered endotracheally. Once intravenous or intraosseous access is obtained, these routes are preferred. Some emergency drugs (i.e., bicarbonate, calcium, and glucose solutions) are not given by the endotracheal route due to the potential for serious damage to the lungs. Most information about endotracheal drug administration in children comes from adult patients, with very few studies addressing pediatric endotracheal drug administration. Studies comparing drug levels after endotracheal versus intravenous delivery of medications show that dosages of medications administered via the endotracheal tube need to be increased in order to obtain effective blood level. Current recommendations for endotracheal medications are to give 2 times the IV dose of atropine, naloxone, and lidocaine; the recommendations for endotracheal doses of epinephrine are to give 10 times the IV dose for children older than 1 month of age and 2 times the dose for neonates. Be sure to use the 1:1,000 concentration of epinephrine for endotracheal drug delivery in infants and children and the 1:10,000 solution for endotracheal drug delivery in neonates (Figure 7-20).

The correct dosage should be confirmed by use of a length-based pediatric resuscitation tape and pediatric drug chart. Add normal saline to obtain a minimum volume of 2 mL for children, compared to 10 mL for adults, in order to deliver enough volume for the medication to flow down the tube and into the trachea.

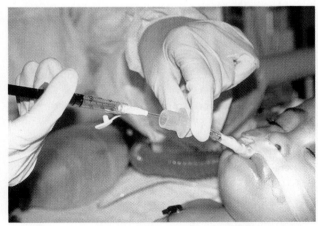

Figure 7-19 Drugs that can be given endotracheally include lidocaine, epinephrine, atropine, and naloxone.

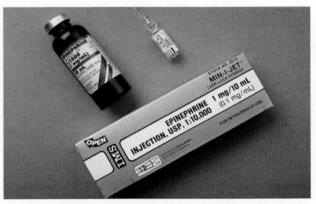

Figure 7-20 Use the 1:1,000 concentration of epinephrine for endotracheal drug delivery in infants and children and the 1:10,000 solution for endotracheal drug delivery in neonates.

Conclusions

Use good basic airway management skills and carefully consider alternative airway management techniques before initiating pediatric endotracheal intubation. A thorough understanding of the indications, the sequence necessary for successful placement, and the methods for confirmation and maintenance of the tube are equally important. Think about possible complications with an eye to prevention, and develop strategies to manage complications as they arise. While no training scenario can adequately simulate an emergency intubation, practice on infant and child manikins and review of procedures are helpful in maintaining skills.

Scenario Review

You were called to the home of an 11-month-old girl. Upon arrival, the mother led you to her bedroom where you found a cyanotic child with very little chest movement. There was vomitus with white powdery fragments on the carpet. The mother told you the child may have swallowed some sleeping pills. You positioned the child's head to open the airway, and suctioned vomitus from the airway. Despite bag-mask ventilation, oxygen saturation shown on the pulse oximeter remained at 85%. Your protocols include endotracheal intubation as an option for management of respiratory failure.

1. *What initial actions would you take to manage this child's airway?*

Many patients will respond to proper positioning, suctioning, and positive pressure ventilation. The presence of vomitus complicated your approach and the airway was suctioned simultaneously with positioning of the patient. You instruct another provider to continue bag-mask ventilation while you prepare the intubation equipment utilizing a length-based resuscitation tape to assist selection of appropriate endotracheal tube sizes. After the tube is placed, a large amount of vomitus is noted in the tube.

2. *How would you determine that your airway management is effective?*

You suction the endotracheal tube to remove the vomitus and then quickly confirm correct placement of the tube by clinical assessment and CO_2 detection. Chest rise is symmetric and there are no gurgling sounds in the stomach. Breath sounds are louder on the right as compared to the left. The 4.5 mm tube is at 16 cm. You realize that the tube should be at the 13 cm mark so you withdraw it until breath sounds are equal. The CO_2 detector is yellow. The tube is in the trachea and is secured with tape. You reassess after securing the tube and pulse oximetry reads 97%. You now consider possible causes of this respiratory arrest, the most likely cause being an overdose. As with many accidental ingestions, prehospital management priorities are supportive. Very few ingestions have antidotes available to field providers. You gather up all the medications within the home and transport the child to the hospital. In the emergency department, tube placement is confirmed and the child is admitted to the pediatric intensive care unit. The child is discharged three days later without complications.

Quick Quiz

1. *Which of the following relies on the body to produce carbon dioxide to assist in the detection of esophageal intubation?*
   - A. Esophageal Detector Device
   - B. Breath sounds bilaterally
   - C. Colorimetric detector
   - D. Sellick maneuver

2. *The endotracheal tube should be advanced until:*
   - A. breath sounds are heard only on the right side of the chest.
   - B. the end of the endotracheal tube is even with the lip.
   - C. the tube is advanced just past the vocal cords.
   - D. another provider advises you to stop.

3. *A benefit of intubation over bag-mask ventilation includes:*
   - A. ability to administer medications.
   - B. less airway trauma.
   - C. better skill retention.
   - D. relative safety of the procedure.

4. *The Sellick maneuver can be useful in:*
   - A. preventing right main stem intubation.
   - B. preventing gastric insufflation.
   - C. administering the appropriate amount of medication via ET tube.
   - D. detecting esophageal intubation.

Glossary

barotrauma　An injury caused by a change in pressure.

cricoid cartilage　The lowermost cartilage of the larynx.

epigastrium　The abdominal area below the sternum.

mainstem bronchus　Either of the two primary divisions of the trachea that lead respectively to the right and left lung.

postictal　A state after a seizure, in which the patient is confused.

vallecula　The space between the base of the tongue and the epiglottis.

Selected References

1. Aijian P. Endotracheal intubation of pediatric patients by paramedics. *Ann Emerg Med.* 1989;18:489–94.

2. Brownstein D, Shugerman R, Cummings P, et al. Prehospital endotracheal intubation of children by paramedics. *Ann Emerg Med.* 1996;28:34–39.

3. Gausche M, Goodrich SM, Poore PD. *Instructor Manual for Advanced Life Support Providers: Pediatric Airway Management Project*; 2nd ed. Torrance, CA: Maternal and Child Health Bureau, National Highway Traffic and Safety Administration, and Agency for Healthcare Research and Quality; 1997. Includes full slide set.

4. Gausche M, Lewis R, Stratton S, et al. Effect of out-of-hospital pediatric endotracheal intubation on survival and neurological outcome. *JAMA.* 2000;283:783–790.

5. Johnston, C. Endotracheal drug delivery. *Pediatr Emerg Care.* 1992:Apr;8(2):94–97.

6. Losek JD, Bonadio WA, Walsh-Kelly C. Prehospital pediatric endotracheal intubation performance review. *Pediatr Emerg Care.* 1989;5:1–4.

7. Nakayama DK, Gardner MJ, Rowe MI. Emergency endotracheal intubation in pediatric trauma. *Ann Surg.* 1990;211:218–223.

8. Pointer JE. Clinical characteristics of paramedics' performance of pediatric endotracheal intubation. *Am J Emerg Med.* 1989;7:364–366.

9. Stratton, SJ, Underwood LA, Whalen SM. Prehospital pediatric endotracheal intubation: A survey of the United States. *Prehosp Disaster Med.* 1993;8:323–326.

10. Tsai A, Kallsen G. Epidemiology of pediatric prehospital care. *Ann Emerg Med.* 1987;16:284–292.

End of Chapter Activities

Technology Resources

Online Course _____

Anatomy Review _____

Online Glossary _____

Web Links _____

Online Quiz _____

Scenarios

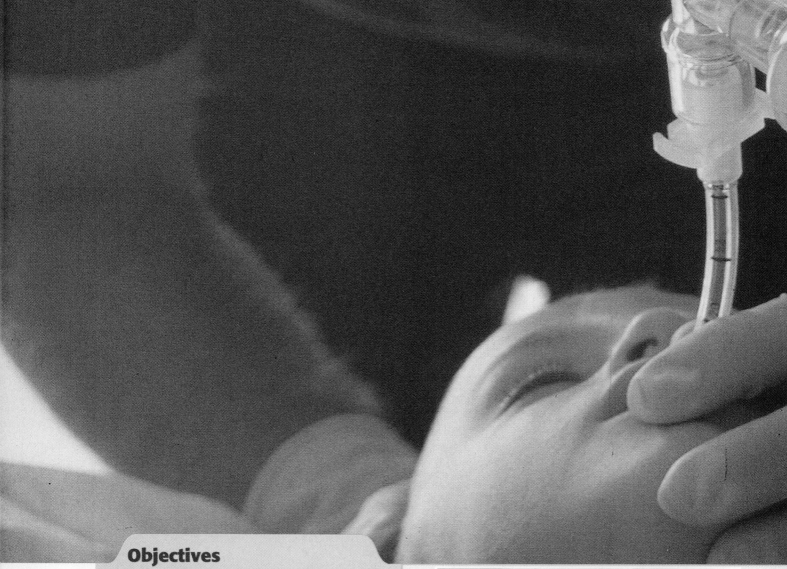

Objectives

1 Discuss the importance of rapid sequence intubation (RSI) in facilitating endotracheal intubation.

2 List the indications and contraindications of alternative forms of airway and respiratory management, including laryngeal mask airway (LMA), needle cricothyrotomy, and use of the gum elastic bougie.

3 Determine the correct size equipment for, and the steps in, the procedures of alternative forms of airway and respiratory management, including laryngeal mask airway, needle cricothyrotomy, and use of the gum elastic bougie.

4 Identify complications in using alternative forms of airway management and determine corrective measures.

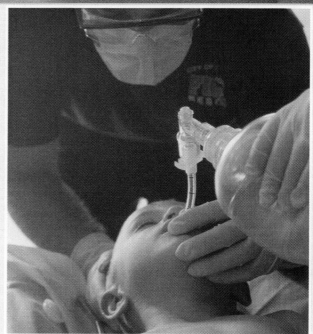

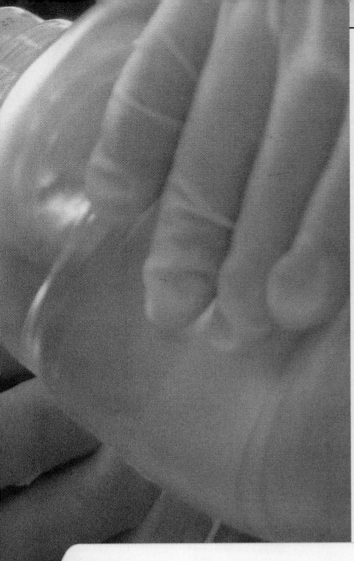

CHAPTER 8

Advanced Techniques in Pediatric Airway Management

Scenario

You are called to the street for an auto versus pedestrian incident. A 10-year-old boy was coming down a hill on his scooter and failed to stop at a crosswalk. Bystanders surround the boy. You begin your assessment and find that the boy is unconscious, has agonal respirations, and his skin is pale. You begin bag-mask ventilation and note chest rise, but ventilation is difficult to maintain because of massive facial injuries. The patient responds to painful stimuli with flexor posturing. Your protocols allow for endotracheal intubation. You are unable to intubate the patient after three attempts.

1. *What are your airway management priorities now?*

2. *What airway techniques could be considered to manage this difficult airway?*

Think about these questions and this case as you read on. We will return to this scenario at the end of the chapter.

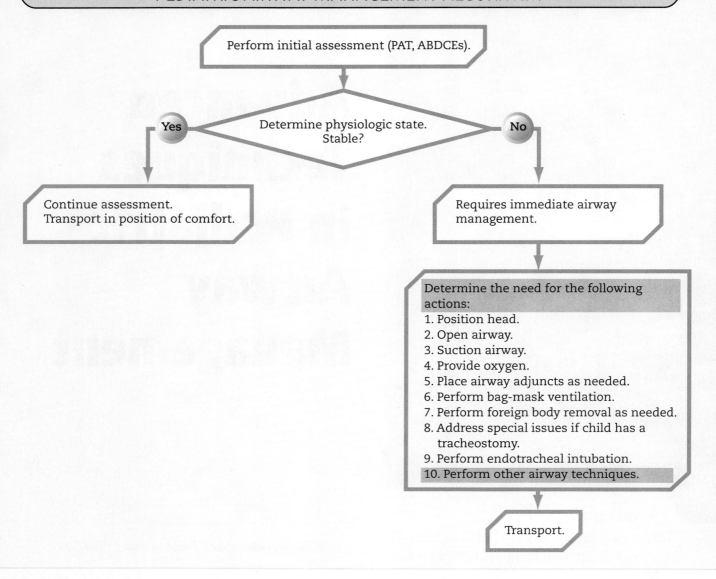

Perform initial assessment (PAT, ABDCEs).

Determine physiologic state. Stable?

Yes → Continue assessment. Transport in position of comfort.

No → Requires immediate airway management.

Determine the need for the following actions:
1. Position head.
2. Open airway.
3. Suction airway.
4. Provide oxygen.
5. Place airway adjuncts as needed.
6. Perform bag-mask ventilation.
7. Perform foreign body removal as needed.
8. Address special issues if child has a tracheostomy.
9. Perform endotracheal intubation.
10. Perform other airway techniques.

Transport.

Introduction

There are limited airway management techniques available to the prehospital provider and yet the field situation can be the most demanding due to patient factors, environmental conditions, lack of personnel, crowd control issues, and potential danger to the providers. Development and practice of strategies to manage the pediatric airway in difficult situations can assist the prehospital provider in problem-solving when the need arises. Basic airway techniques, such as the use of airway adjuncts to maintain an open airway passage and bag-mask ventilation to maintain ventilation and oxygenation, should be used in initial management of these cases. If these basic maneuvers fail, then additional methods may be needed to manage the difficult airway.

This chapter will review advanced techniques in the management of the pediatric airway. Techniques such as the use of the gum elastic bougie and rapid sequence intubation can facilitate endotracheal intubation, whereas cricothyrotomy and laryngeal mask airway are considered rescue techniques if intubation is unsuccessful.

Gum Elastic Bougie

The gum elastic bougie, or tracheal tube introducer (Figure 8-1), was first described in 1949 by MacIntosh as an aid to endotracheal intubation for patients 14 years of age or older. Essentially, it is a long stylet made of woven polyester and covered with resin (Eschmann stylet). A plastic version of the endotracheal tube introducer (GreenField Medical Sourcing, Inc., Northborough, MA) has been produced and shown to be useful in facilitating intubation.

Where's the Evidence?

Gum Elastic Bougie

There are no published studies of the gum elastic bougie used by paramedics in a field setting. There is a study evaluating the ability of paramedics to use the device on a manikin in a simulated difficult airway situation. Thirty-five paramedics, experienced in endotracheal intubation, attending a recertification course were asked to participate in the study. All paramedics received a brief 5-minute didactic session on the use of the tracheal tube introducer. Paramedics were then asked to intubate an adult manikin using standard techniques and the tracheal tube introducer. The success rate was 34/35 (97%) for standard laryngoscopy, endotracheal intubation, and use of the tracheal tube introducer.

Several randomized controlled trials of the gum elastic bougie have been reported in the anesthesia literature. Gataure and colleagues showed in a simulated difficult airway in a manikin that the gum elastic bougie was used successfully to place the endotracheal tube in 96% of the cases compared to 66% of cases using standard techniques. This result was highly significant and authors concluded that the gum elastic bougie should be available for use by anesthesiologists to manage a difficult airway. Nolan

and Wilson evaluated the use of the gum elastic bougie in facilitating endotracheal intubation in 157 routine surgery patients with a simulated cervical spine injury. Visualization of the cords was limited in 45% of patients, and in 22% of the group nothing could be seen beyond the epiglottis. Seventy-nine patients were randomized to standard techniques and 78 to the gum elastic bougie. There were five intubation failures (6%) in the standard group and none in the gum elastic bougie group. In addition, all of the five patients in the standard intubation failure group were successfully intubated using the gum elastic bougie.

1. Le DH, Reed DB, Weinstein G, et al. Paramedic use of endotracheal tube introducers for the difficult airway. *Prehosp Emerg Care.* 2002;5:155–158.

2. Moscati R, Jehle D, Christiansen G, et al. Endotracheal tube introducer for failed intubations: A variant of the gum elastic bougie. *Ann Emerg Med.* 2000;36:52–56.

3. Nocera A. A flexible solution for emergency intubation difficulties. *Ann Emerg Med.* 1996;27:665–667.

4. Nolan JP, Wilson ME. Orotracheal intubation in patients with potential cervical spine injuries. An indication for the gum elastic bougie. *Anesthesia.* 1993;48:630–633.

5. Pitt K, Woollard M. Should paramedics bougie on down? *Pre-Hosp Immediate Care.* 2000;4:68–70. http://www.asancep.org.uk/ShouldParamedicBougieonDown.htm. Accessed February 20, 2004.

Anatomical Considerations

video Anatomical considerations when using a gum elastic bougie include:

- The larynx is anterior to the epiglottis.
- The tracheal rings are stiff and made of cartilage.

The gum elastic bougie works based on two important principles: 1) the airway is anterior to the epiglottis; and 2) the tracheal rings are stiff and made of cartilage, while the esophagus is smooth. The tip of the gum elastic bougie points anteriorly and can be directed into the airway (Figure 8-2). The stiffness of

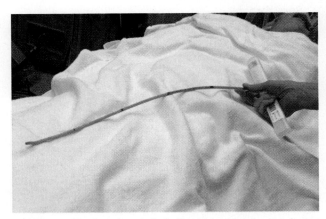

Figure 8-1 Gum elastic bougie for facilitating endotracheal intubation in adolescents or adults.

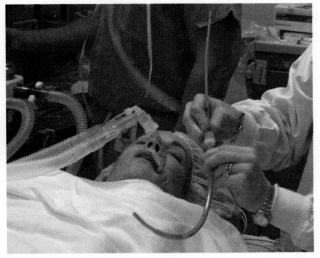

Figure 8-2 The tip of the gum elastic bougie points anteriorly and can be directed into the airway.

the tracheal rings in adolescent and adult patients causes a click as the gum elastic bougie impacts them; the smooth esophagus does not. This has been shown to be a reliable sign of correct placement of the gum elastic bougie except in young children. In younger children the tracheal rings are not calcified, making it difficult to feel the tracheal rings as the gum elastic bougie passes over them.

Indications

Indications for using a gum elastic bougie are as follows:
- Inability to visualize the cords
- Inability to intubate using standard techniques

Standard intubation techniques should be tried first, as studies have shown that standard techniques are at least 10 seconds faster than the gum elastic bougie technique. The gum elastic bougie should be performed in cases of failed intubation or an inability to adequately visualize the airway. This technique is used more extensively in Europe than in the United States.

Contraindications

Contraindications for using a gum elastic bougie include:
- Pediatric patients younger than 14 years of age

Procedure Step-by-Step

video The steps for using a gum elastic bougie are as follows:
1. Remove the gum elastic bougie from the packaging.
2. Place the lubricated end of the endotracheal tube over the straight end of the stylet.

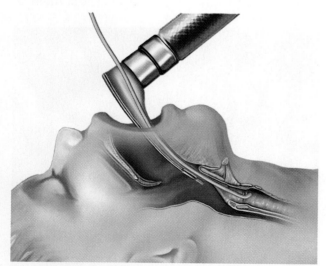

Figure 8-3 After inserting the laryngoscope and visualizing the epiglottis, insert the flexed end of the gum elastic bougie slightly beyond and upward through the vocal cords.

3. Insert the laryngoscope and visualize the epiglottis.
4. Insert the flexed end of the gum elastic bougie slightly beyond and upward through the cords (Figure 8-3).
5. Continue advancing the gum elastic bougie until clicks are felt, indicating the tracheal rings.
6. Slide the lubricated tube down the gum elastic bougie and through the cords.
7. If resistance is felt, rotate the endotracheal tube 90° counterclockwise so that the bevel faces posteriorly.
8. Remove the laryngoscope and then withdraw the gum elastic bougie.
9. Assess for correct endotracheal tube placement and secure the endotracheal tube.

TRICKS
of the Trade

- Be sure the tip of the gum elastic bougie points upward in a "J" shape.
- To insert the device, it is best to visualize at least the epiglottis and ideally the arytenoids cartilages.
- If resistance to passage of the gum elastic bougie is felt, it is possible that it is resting at the carina. Withdraw it 3–5 cm.
- Passage of the endotracheal tube can be difficult at times. Consider using a half to full size smaller as there may be laryngeal edema. Also, if there is resistance in passage of the tube, rotate the tube counterclockwise slightly and attempt to reinsert.

Complications

Complications of using a gum elastic bougie include the following:
- Damage to trachea or esophagus
- Sore throat
- Hoarseness

Reported complications of the use of this device are rare. This device should not be used in children younger than 14 years of age.

■ Rapid Sequence Intubation

video Rapid sequence intubation or induction (RSI) is a technique that facilitates success of intubation. It involves the use of medication that sedates and paralyzes the patient. These medications can reduce the physiological effects of intubation on heart rate, blood pressure, and intracranial pressure. RSI has been shown in the emergency department to increase suc-

Where's the Evidence?

Rapid Sequence Intubation

Wayne and colleagues performed a retrospective review of 1,657 consecutive patients age 16 years or older receiving prehospital succinylcholine administered by paramedics. Success rates for intubation were reported at 95.5%. The esophageal intubation rate was 0.3%.

Brownstein et al reviewed prehospital endotracheal intubation in 654 children in Seattle, Washington. Only 355 records (54%) were complete enough to review. Succinylcholine was used to facilitate intubation in 47% of patients. Overall complications occurred in 24% of patients: 34 patients with mainstem bronchus intubation (13%), 15 with aspiration (6%), 9 with pneumothorax (3%), 5 with unrecognized esophageal intubation (2%), and 2 with oral/dental trauma (1%).

Sing and colleagues reviewed the use of succinylcholine in 40 pediatric patients requiring intubation by flight paramedics. The success rate was 97.5%. Intubation mishaps occurred in 13 patients (33%): 9 patients with multiple attempts (23%), 8 with aspiration (20%), and 1 with esophageal intubation (3%). Bradycardia occurred in 3 patients (8%).

Mizelle and colleagues recently reported a series of three cases in which RSI was inappropriately used in the field setting leading to anoxic injury with severe neurological deficits or death. These investigators cited lack of training, poor clinical judgment, and failure to use airway rescue devices as the causes for these outcomes.

Although McDonald and Bailey report that 29 states (58%) use neuromuscular blocking agents to facilitate intubation in the prehospital setting, only 18 states use these agents delivered by ground crews, of which 11 are exclusively paramedic and 7 include a registered nurse on the crew.

None of the studies to date have systematically evaluated the use of RSI as compared to bag-mask ventilation, nor have they evaluated the effect of RSI on patient outcome.

1. Brownstein D, Shugerman R, Cummings P, et al. Prehospital endotracheal intubation of children by paramedics. *Ann Emerg Med.* 1996;28(1):34–39.

2. McDonald CC, Bailey B. Out-of-hospital use of neuromuscular-blocking agents in the United States. *Prehosp Emerg Care.* 1998; 2:29–32.

3. Mizelle HL, Rothrock SG, Silvestri S, Pagane J. Preventable morbidity and mortality from prehospital paralytic assisted intubation: Can we expect outcomes comparable to hospital-based practice? *Prehosp Emerg Care.* 2002;6:472–475.

4. Sing RF, Reilly PM, Rotondo MF, et al. Out-of-hospital rapid-sequence induction for intubation of the pediatric patient. *Acad Emerg Med.* 1997;4:80–81.

5. Wayne MA, Friedland E. Prehospital use of succinylcholine: A 20-year review. *Prehosp Emerg Care.* 1999;3:107–109.

cess of intubation and reduce complications of the procedure. It has been in use in the United States in the prehospital setting since 1972, although the first cases reported in the literature were in 1988. Since this time, many prehospital case reports and case series have been published. Most of these studies have been performed in air medical systems with some notable exceptions.

Anatomical Considerations

video The anatomical considerations for rapid sequence intubation are the same as for endotracheal intubation discussed in Chapter 7: Endotracheal Intubation.

Indications

Indications for rapid sequence intubation include the following:
- Facilitate intubation in a patient who is difficult to intubate without paralysis
- Head trauma patient in need of hyperventilation

Contraindications

Contraindications to rapid sequence intubation include the following:
- Abnormal airway anatomy (i.e., major facial trauma)
- Upper airway obstruction
- Laryngeal fracture

Procedure Step-by-Step

video The steps for performing rapid sequence intubation are described below and in Skill Drill 8-1.
1. Prepare equipment and medications. The mnemonic S-O-A-P-ME has been used by health professionals to remember the equipment and medications needed for rapid sequence intubation.
   - **S**uction (assume patient has a full stomach)
   - **O**xygen
   - **A**irway equipment:
     - Oral and nasal airways
     - Bag-mask devices and masks

- Endotracheal tubes and stylets
  - ♦ Endotracheal tubes - two sizes available; appropriate size based on length or other calculation and 1/2 size smaller
- Laryngoscope handles and blades
- Magill forceps
- **P**harmacology (**Table 8-1**):
  - Atropine
  - Lidocaine
  - Sedatives
  - Neuromuscular blocking agents
- **M**onitoring Equipment:
  - Cardiorespiratory monitor/pulse oximeter
  - End-tidal CO_2 detector or monitor

2. Place patient on cardiac monitor and pulse oximeter. Monitoring the patient's heart rate and oxygen saturation are critical to the safe use of RSI medications.

3. Ensure that all necessary airway equipment is functional and available. The steps taken to prepare the equipment are the same as in preparation of intubation without RSI (**Figure 8-4**).

4. Place an intravenous line (IV) or intraosseous line (IO). IV lines are preferred, but an IO line could be used if IV placement is unsuccessful.

5. Determine dosage of all RSI medications. Calculation of drug doses of medication based on weight is subject to error, especially when a patient is critically ill and time for the delivery of medications is limited. The safest way to determine accurate dosing of medication is to use the length-based resuscitation tape. The procedure for use of the tape is discussed in Chapter 2: Assessment.

6. Administer sedative and atropine. Atropine is used in children to prevent the bradycardia that may occur with stimulation of the poste-

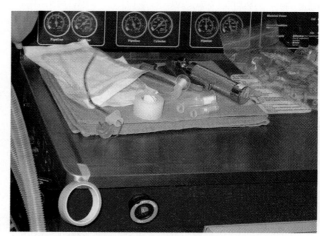

Figure 8-4 Prepare equipment for intubation.

Table 8-1:	Medications for Use in Prehospital RSI		
Medication	Purpose	Dose	Important Side Effects
Etomidate	Sedate	0.3 mg/kg IV	May cause vomiting
Diazepam	Sedate	0.2 mg/kg IV or IO	May cause respiratory depression; duration of action is long
Midazolam	Sedate	0.1 mg/kg IV, IM, or IO	May cause respiratory depression; duration of action is short
Atropine	Prevent bradycardia	0.02 mg/kg IV, IM, or IO 0.1 mg minimum dose; max single dose 0.5 mg for child; 1.0 mg for adolescent	
Lidocaine	Prevents rise in ICP (use only with head trauma)	1 mg/kg IV or IO	Can cause hypotension if pushed rapidly
Rocuronium	Paralyze	1 mg/kg IV	Effects seen in 30–60 sec; duration of blockade 25–60 min; may cause increase in heart rate
Succinylcholine	Paralyze	2 mg/kg IV, IM, or IO	Effects in 15–30 sec; duration of action 3–5 min; DO NOT use in patients with prior history of paralysis (injury, muscular dystrophy, or cerebral palsy) or conditions which may cause high potassium values such as renal (kidney) failure

rior pharynx (back of the throat) with intubation. Atropine is not needed in children greater than 10 years of age or adults. Atropine is not given routinely prior to pediatric intubation in some EMS systems, but it should always be available and ready for use if bradycardia ensues. It is given routinely prior to pediatric intubation in emergency departments. The sedative is used to decrease the anxiety and discomfort associated with intubation. This is extremely important because patients who are fully aware of the intubation are frightened.

7. Administer succinylcholine. Succinylcholine takes one to two minutes before the effect of the drug is seen. Patients may show muscle fasciculations or muscle twitching when the drug takes effect. This reaction occurs because the drug is causing muscle contraction throughout the body. You may not see this effect as readily in infants and small children because of the small amount of total body muscle mass. Wait about one minute after drug administration before attempting intubation.

Side effects of succinylcholine can be life threatening. Although very rare, malignant hyperthermia, a condition of unstable temperature and cardiovascular control, may cause death. Another possible reaction occurs in patients who have had long standing paralysis. In these patients, the muscles are sensitized over time and with contraction may release large amounts of potassium into the blood stream. Any patient with acute paralysis will not have this reaction as the sensitization of the muscle occurs over days to weeks. In the pediatric age group, the patients who may have this reaction are those with muscular dystrophy, cerebral palsy, or other neurological injury. Caution should be exercised in giving succinylcholine to patients with potentially high potassium values in the blood, such as patients with renal (kidney) failure, since administration of succinylcholine results in an additional rise in potassium and may push potassium levels into the toxic range. Toxic potassium levels can lead to serious cardiac dysfunction and death.

8. Perform endotracheal intubation. The procedure for intubation is the same as outlined in Chapter 7: Endotracheal Intubation. Careful patient monitoring is necessary to quickly identify complications of the procedure or side effects of the medication delivered. Once the placement of the tube has been confirmed (clinically and with CO_2 detection), the tube is secured.

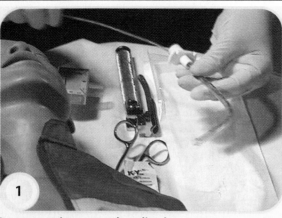

1

Prepare equipment and medications.
Ensure that all necessary airway equipment is functional and available.

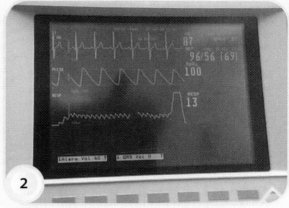

2

Place the patient on a cardiac monitor and pulse oximeter (if available).

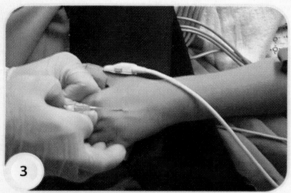

3

Place an intravenous line (IV) or intraosseous line (IO).

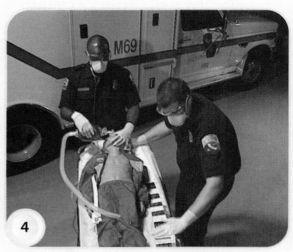

4

Determine the dosage of all RSI medications.

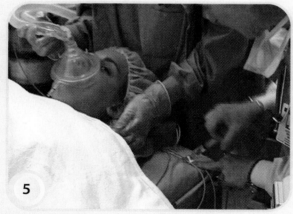

5

Administer sedative and atropine (as appropriate).
Administer succinylcholine.

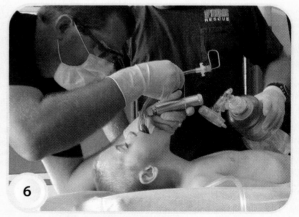

6

Perform endotracheal intubation.

If you are unable to intubate the patient, begin bag-mask ventilation. Place an airway adjunct as needed to keep the airway open. Succinylcholine will last about 6 minutes so the patient's ventilation will have to be assisted until the patient is able to adequately breathe on his or her own. Patients in cardiorespiratory arrest have decreased tone and should be able to be intubated without RSI.

Complications

Complications of rapid sequence intubation include the following:

- Esophageal intubation
- Mainstem bronchus intubation
- Vomiting and aspiration
- Incorrect endotracheal tube size determination
- Hypoxia
- Endotracheal tube dislodgement
- Trauma to the mouth or airway structures
- Related to succinylcholine: bradycardia, increase in potassium blood level, malignant hyperthermia

Corrective maneuvers for the above complications are discussed in Chapter 7: Endotracheal Intubation. The key to the treatment of all complications is early recognition. Most of these complications can be detected immediately with appropriate monitoring techniques and then corrective maneuvers initiated. Vomiting may be treated by suctioning and placing patient in the left lateral decubitus position to avoid aspiration. The bradycardia associated with succinylcholine use can be prevented with pretreatment of atropine. The increase in potassium may be avoided by appropriate history taking, if possible, prior to administration of RSI medications. If not, patient will show electrocardiographic signs of hyperkalemia (increased potassium levels in the blood), which include peaking of T waves followed by a widening of the QRS complex (Figure 8-5) or the patient may develop a dysrhythmia and cardiopulmonary arrest. Immediate treatment of hyperkalemia involves administration of calcium chloride, which will protect the heart from the effects

of potassium and/or sodium bicarbonate, which causes potassium to shift from extracellular to intracellular fluids. Do not put these drugs in the same line or they will result in precipitation. Field treatment of malignant hyperthermia includes appropriate monitoring and cooling measures. Patients with any of the signs of a reaction to succinylcholine should be rapidly transported to the emergency department with corrective measures en route.

Laryngeal Mask Airway

Introduction

video The laryngeal mask airway (LMA) is a device that consists of a large bore tube with a distal inflatable molded mask placed above the laryngeal inlet to direct gases into the lungs (Figure 8-6). Once the cuff on the mask is inflated, it makes a relatively airtight seal over the larynx. It does not prevent aspiration of gastric contents, but few reports of aspiration occur in the literature. A bag-mask device can be connected to the tube end of the LMA and squeezed to achieve chest rise. Currently, only three sizes are available in disposable form (3, 4, and 5), none of which are appropriate for infants or small children; however, disposable forms may become available. There are reusable LMAs available in sizes 1, 1.5, 2, and 2.5 but they require special cleaning prior to reuse, which makes their use less feasible in the prehospital setting (Figure 8-7).

The device was first introduced by Brain in 1983. Since this time, the LMA (LMA North America, Inc.) had been used extensively in anesthesia, often replacing bag-mask ventilation for airway management. Recently there has been more literature published on the use of this device in prehospital and emergency department settings in the United States. There are a variety of reports on the use of the LMA in Europe.

Anatomical Considerations

video Anatomical considerations when using a laryngeal mask airway include the following:

- The floppy and U-shaped epiglottis can fold over, leading to suboptimal positioning of the LMA.

Overall anatomical differences in adults and children play a smaller role with the insertion of the LMA than with endotracheal intubation.

Indications

Indications for using a laryngeal mask airway include:

- Patients in whom bag-mask ventilation or endotracheal intubation fails

At this point, the role of LMA in the prehospital setting is ill-defined. It has been used to successfully manage the airway in cases of neonatal resuscitation and in adult patients in cardiopulmonary arrest, but

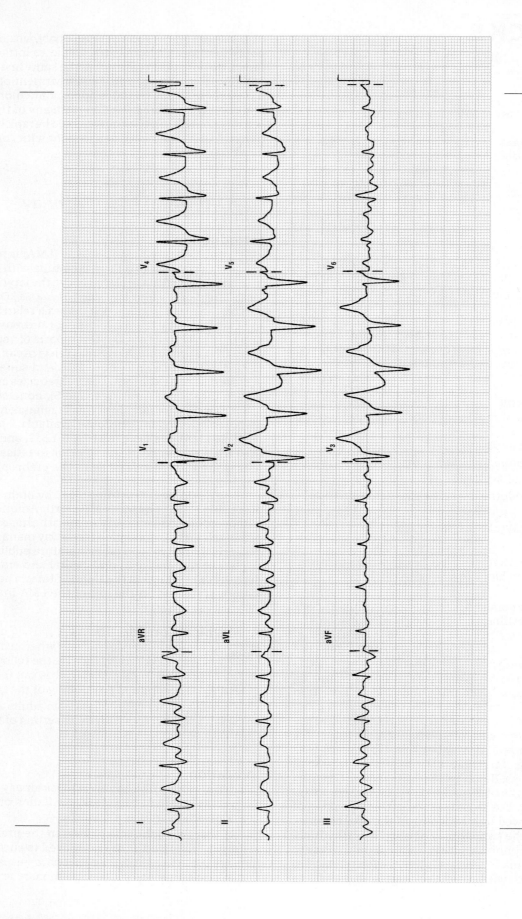

Figure 8-5 Widening of QRS complex may indicate hyperkalemia.

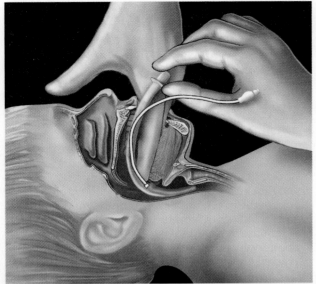

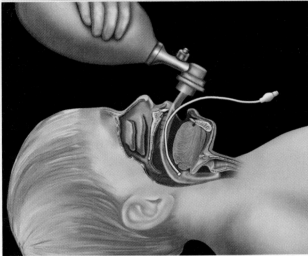

Figure 8-6 The laryngeal mask airway (LMA) is a device that consists of a large bore tube with a distal inflatable molded mask placed above the laryngeal inlet to direct gases into the lungs.

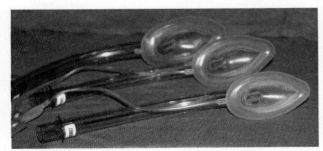

Figure 8-7 Laryngeal mask airways.

to date there is sparse information on its use in emergency settings for airway management of children. Theoretically, LMA may be more ideal for management of the pediatric airway in the prehospital setting than either bag-mask ventilation or endotracheal intubation because of the ease of teaching the technique, the small amount of equipment required to perform the procedure, and the speed to which the LMA can be inserted. Reports of aspiration are rare and complications associated with endotracheal intubation such as esophageal intubation or mainstem bronchus intubation are avoided by use of the LMA. Field studies evaluating its use on patients need to be performed to fully define the indications for its use in this setting.

Contraindications

Contraindications for using a laryngeal mask airway include the following:

- Awake patients or patients with a gag reflex
- Patients requiring high pressures to ventilate

Contraindications for the use of this device are few, but center around two concerns: 1) the fact that the LMA is a low pressure seal and it may be difficult to ventilate patients who require high pressures to ventilate (asthma, submersion [near drowning]); and 2) the LMA does not fully protect the airway from regurgitated stomach contents as can occur in non-fasted patients (emergency patients) or those that have delayed gastric emptying (obesity and pregnancy).

Procedure Step-by-Step

video The steps for using an LMA are described below and in **Skill Drill 8-2**.

1. Place the patient in the sniffing position.
2. Organize the equipment for the procedure.
   - LMAs of all sizes
   - Water-soluble lubricant
   - Syringe
3. Determine the size of the laryngeal mask based on the **Table 8-2**.
4. Deflate the cuff of the LMA so that it forms a smooth spoon shape while compressing the diaphragm portion against a flat surface.
5. Lubricate the LMA with a water-soluble lubricant.
6. Hold the LMA like a pen, with the index finger placed at the junction of the cuff and the tube.
7. Insert the LMA into the mouth and flatten the diaphragm portion against the hard palate.
8. Continue to press the LMA against the hard palate past the tongue, pushing toward the head (upward) with an index finger and stop when resistance is felt.

9. Inflate the cuff until the LMA protrudes slightly (see **Table 8-2** for inflation volumes).

10. Attach manual resuscitator and begin ventilation. Look for chest rise.

11. A soft gauze bite block can be used to protect the LMA from the patient's teeth.

Table 8-2: LMA Sizes and Cuff Volume by Patient Weight

Size of LMA	Weight (kg)	Air Volume for Cuff (mL)
1	< 5kg (Neonate)	4
1.5	5–10 (Infants)	7
2.0	10–20 (Infants and children)	10
2.5	20–30 (Children)	14
3	30–50 (Children and adolescents)	20
4	50–70 (Small adults)	30
5	70–100 (Normal to large adults)	40
6	>100 (Large adults)	50

Where's the Evidence?

Endotracheal Intubation vs. Laryngeal Mask Placement

Pennant and Walker compared the ability of paramedics to perform endotracheal intubation versus laryngeal mask placement on 40 healthy anesthetized adults in an operating room setting. Ninety-four percent of the students were able to place the LMA successfully on the first attempt and only 69% were able to intubate the trachea on the first attempt. Five students were unable to intubate the trachea after 3 attempts, whereas none of the students were unable to place the LMA. Adequate ventilation was achieved significantly sooner with the LMA (39 seconds) versus endotracheal intubation (88 seconds).

Rumball and MacDonald report on the study of the Pharyngeal Tracheal Lumen Airway (PTL), the LMA, the esophageal tracheal Combitube on adult patients requiring airway management in the prehospital setting. The success rate for placement of the LMA was 73% and 3 patients had vomiting and possible aspiration of stomach contents. The complication rate of LMA insertion in the prehospital setting is yet to be determined, but Brimacombe and Berry report an aspiration rate of 2 cases per 10,000 patients when LMAs are used in the operating room.

There are a few case reports of LMAs being successful in the prehospital setting for young infants but there are no major studies of its use by paramedics to support ventilation in children in this setting to date.

1. Berry AM, Brimacombe JR, Verghase C. The laryngeal mask airway in emergency medicine, neonatal resuscitation, and intensive care medicine. *Int Anesthesiol Clin.* 1998;36:91–109.

2. Brimacombe JR, Berry A. The incidence of aspiration associated with the laryngeal mask airway: A meta-analysis of published literature. *J Clin Anesth.* 1995;7:297–305.

3. Idris AA, Gabriellai A. Advances in airway management. *Emerg Clin N Am.* 2002;20:843–857.

4. Pennant JH, Walker MB. Comparison of the endotracheal tube and laryngeal mask in airway management by paramedical personnel. *Anesth Analg.* 1992;74:531–534.

5. Rumball CJ, MacDonald D. The PTL, Combitube, laryngeal mask, and oral airway: A randomized prehospital comparative study of ventilatory device effectiveness and cost-effectiveness in 470 cases of cardiorespiratory arrest. *Prehosp Emerg Care.* 1997;1:1–10.

6. Sasada MP, Gabbott DA. The role of laryngeal mask airway in prehospital care. *Resuscitation.* 1994;28:97–102.

7. Tanigawa K, Shigematsu A. Choice of airway devices for 12,020 cases of nontraumatic cardiac arrest in Japan. *Prehosp Emerg Care.* 1998;2:96–100.

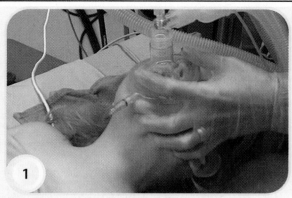

Place the patient in the sniffing position.

Organize the equipment for the procedure: LMAs of all sizes, water-soluble lubricant, and a syringe.

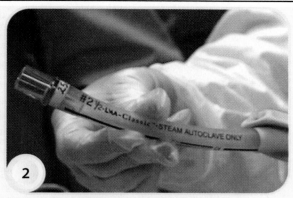

Determine the size of the laryngeal mask.

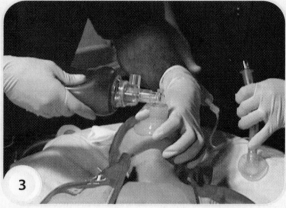

Deflate the cuff of the LMA so that it forms a smooth spoon shape while compressing the diaphragm portion against a flat surface.

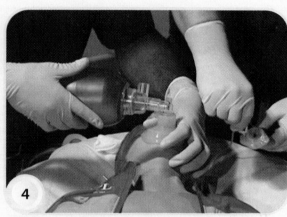

Lubricate the LMA with a water-soluble lubricant.

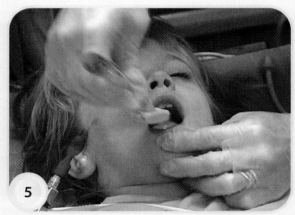

Hold the LMA like a pen, with the index finger placed at the junction of the cuff and the tube.

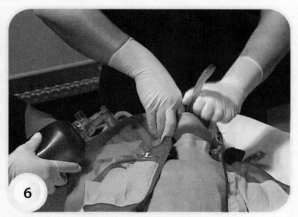

Insert the LMA into the mouth and flatten the diaphragm portion against the hard palate.

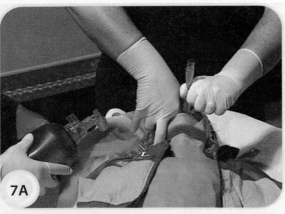

7A

Continue to press the LMA against the hard palate past the tongue, pushing toward the head (upward) with an index finger. Stop when you feel resistance (A).

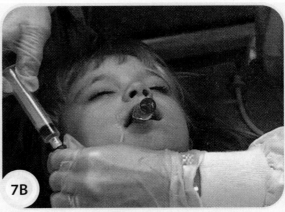

7B

Inflate the cuff until the LMA protrudes slightly (B).

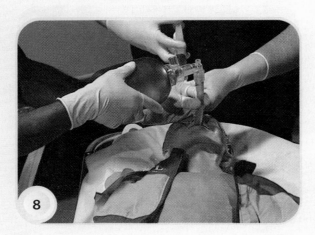

8

Attach the manual resuscitator and begin ventilation. Look for chest rise.

A soft gauze bite block can be used to protect the LMA from the patient's teeth.

TRICKS of the Trade

- Note that failure to press the diaphragm portion of the LMA against the hard palate can cause the end to fold back on itself and prevent further insertion. If so, remove and begin again.
- The curved portion of the LMA should be pointing toward the patient and away from health care provider. Note that a black line is located on the surface of the LMA to aid in confirming correct positioning; if you are standing at the head of the patient looking down to the patient's feet, the black line should be facing you (Figure 8-8).

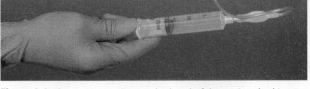

Figure 8-8 If you are standing at the head of the patient looking toward the patient's feet, the black line on the LMA should be facing you.

Complications

Complications when using a laryngeal mask airway include the following:

- Hypoxemia
- Vomiting
- Aspiration of gastric contents

Vomiting and aspiration are uncommon. If vomiting occurs, the patient may be placed in the left lateral decubitus position and the airway and stomach suctioned.

Hypoxemia may be prevented by reducing the length of attempts of insertion to 30 seconds and providing bag-mask ventilation between attempts.

Needle Cricothyrotomy

Introduction

Needle cricothyrotomy is a technique that involves the placement of a needle or catheter into the cricothyroid membrane to bypass the upper airway and instill oxygen into the trachea. Ventilation through the small diameter is limited or nonexistent. This technique has been utilized when standard airway techniques (bag-mask ventilation, endotracheal intubation) fail. Often the patient settings are upper airway obstruction, massive facial trauma, severe anaphylaxis, or oropharyngeal hemorrhage. This technique can be used in any age child but supporting evidence for its use is lacking. There is some data on the open surgical technique for cricothyrotomy but this technique may not be appropriate for children under six years of age.

Anatomical Considerations

video Anatomical considerations when performing a needle cricothyrotomy include:

- The narrowest portion of the pediatric airway, the cricothyroid membrane (Figure 8-9).

   This anatomical difference makes the performance of the open surgical technique more risky. The major concern is laceration of major vessels that lie next to the cricothyroid membrane. The percutaneous approach may be the best alternative for the younger children. Because the narrowest portion of the airway in children is the cricothyroid membrane, there is a risk that a foreign body could become lodged at that level, which could make needle cricothyrotomy difficult or unsuccessful in bypassing the obstruction.

Indications

Indications for performing needle cricothyrotomy include the following:

- Upper airway obstruction if the obstruction cannot otherwise be removed
- Airway rescue technique if endotracheal intubation or LMA cannot be performed

   Because there is so little information available about the use of this procedure in the field on adults and children, defining indications and contraindications is mostly theoretical.

Contraindications

Contraindications to performing a needle cricothyrotomy include the following:
- Successful management of the airway by alternate means including bag-mask ventilation, LMA, or endotracheal intubation.
- Fractures of the larynx

Where's the Evidence?

Surgical and Needle Cricothryotomy

There is very little data on the use of needle cricothyrotomy in the field. Johnson and colleagues evaluated a percutaneous (through the skin) device to perform needle cricothyrotomy versus the open surgical technique of a surgical cricothyrotomy (an incision is made in the patient's neck with a scalpel) on cadavers. Success rates for the two procedures performed by 44 paramedic students were not significantly different. Authors also found that the open surgical technique was faster and easier to perform than when using a commercially available needle cricothyrotomy kit. This may not be true for all commercially available kits.

Spaite and Maralee reported on 20 patients who received surgical cricothyrotomy in the prehospital setting. Two of these patients were children (11 years and 15 years). The procedure was attempted in 16 of 20 patients (80%) meeting the indications for the procedure and was successful in 14 of those patients (88%). Complications occurred in 31% of patients including two patients in which the procedure could not be performed.

Robinson and colleagues report on 12 years of experience in performing surgical cricothyrotomy by nurses or physicians as part of an aeromedical program. During the 12 years of the study, 8,833 patients were transported, 1,589 required intubation (18%), and of these patients, 8 required cricothyrotomy (0.5%). Cricothyrotomy was successful in five of eight patients (63%). The authors concluded that training practices for this procedure need reevaluation.

1. Robinson KJ, Katz R, Jacobs LM. A 12-year experience with prehospital cricothyrotomies. *Air Med J.* 2002;20:27–30.
2. Spaite DW, Maralee J. Prehospital cricothyrotomy: An investigation of indications, technique, complications, and patient outcome. *Ann Emerg Med.* 1990;19:279–285.

Procedure Step-by-Step

video The steps for performing a needle cricothyrotomy are described below and in Skill Drill 8-3.
1. Identify the cricothyroid membrane.
2. Locate and puncture the cricothyroid membrane using a 12- to 14-gauge over-the-needle catheter or a commercially available kit.
3. Use a syringe to draw back air to confirm position as you enter the trachea.
4. Aim the needle at a 45° angle toward the child's feet and slip the catheter over the needle and into the wound. A modification of this technique involves a wire inserted into the tra-

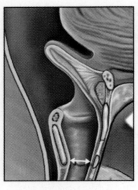
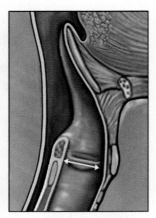

Narrowest portion of pediatric airway = cricoid

Narrowest portion of adult airway = vocal cords

Figure 8-9 The cricothyroid membrane.

chea, followed by a dilator and then a 3.0 mm endotracheal tube threaded over the wire, or placement of a commercially available device.

5. Ventilation by this technique is limited but the patient can be oxygenated; a 3.0 mm adaptor can be placed on the end of the catheter.

6. Attach a manual resuscitator. This may not be as good as an actual jet ventilator.

Complications

Complications when performing a needle cricothyrotomy include the following:

- Failure to complete the procedure successfully
- Hemorrhage
- Thyroid cartilage fracture
- Infection
- Air in the mediastinum or subcutaneous emphysema (air in soft tissues)

It is unclear how frequently these complications are encountered in the field setting as there are no studies available which systematically evaluate the success and complication rate of needle cricothyrotomy in children. Confirming the location of cricothyroid membrane, using good technique, aspirating air prior to insertion of the catheter, and attempting ventilation will help to avoid these complications.

skill drill 8-3: Needle Cricothyrotomy

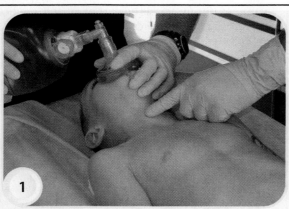

1 Identify the cricothyroid membrane.

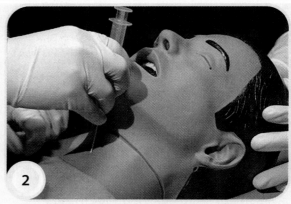

2 Locate and puncture the cricothyroid membrane using a 12- to 14-gauge over-the-needle catheter or a commercially available kit.

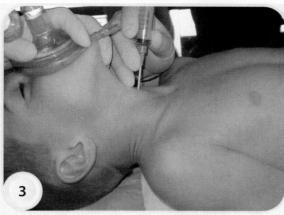

3 Use a syringe to draw back air to confirm position as you enter the trachea.

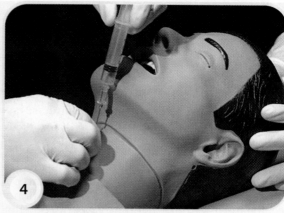

4 Aim the needle at a 45° angle toward the child's feet and slip the catheter over the needle and into the wound.

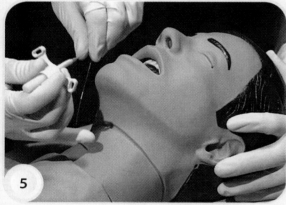

5 A modification of this technique involves a wire inserted into the trachea, followed by a dilator and then a 3.0 mm endotracheal tube threaded over the wire or placement of a commercially available device.

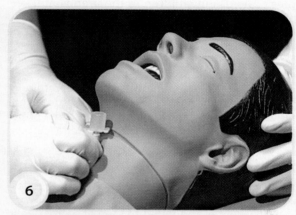

6 Ventilation by this technique is limited but the patient can be oxygenated; a 3.0 mm adaptor can be placed on the end of the catheter.

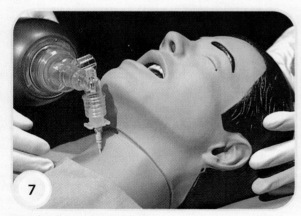

7 Attach a manual resuscitator.

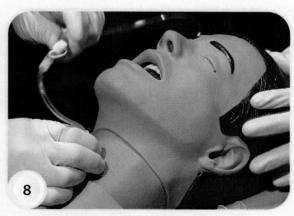

8 This may not be as good as an actual jet ventilator.

Conclusions

The gum elastic bougie may help to facilitate intubation in adolescents and young adults, but should not be used in young children.

RSI has been shown to increase the overall success of intubation and possibly reduce complication rates, but very little data is available on the effect of the procedure to improve outcome. Careful assessment is necessary to ensure that RSI is not used inappropriately on patients who do not require support of ventilation.

The LMA has great potential for use in the prehospital setting, but there are some limitations and potential complications because the airway does not protect the trachea from aspiration of gastric contents. More data, especially with children, is needed to define the role of LMA in prehospital airway management.

Needle cricothyrotomy is a procedure that is used when all other airway techniques fail. There are no studies of its use in children in the prehospital setting. Almost all pediatric patients can be managed with bag-mask ventilation; the one exception may be airway obstruction, and it is in this type of emergency setting that needle cricothyrotomy may be used. The safety of this procedure is unknown.

Basic airway management is the cornerstone of prehospital airway management. More studies are needed to evaluate the use of alternate forms of pediatric airway management in the prehospital setting.

Scenario Review

You were called to the street for an auto versus pedestrian incident. A 10-year-old boy was coming down a hill on his scooter and failed to stop at a crosswalk. You noted that the boy was unconscious, had agonal respirations, and pale skin. You began bag-mask ventilation and noted chest rise, but ventilation was difficult to maintain because of massive facial injuries. The patient responded to painful stimuli with flexor posturing. You were unable to intubate the patient after three attempts.

1. *What are your airway management priorities now?*

This is a difficult airway situation. Management priorities include establishment of an open airway. An oropharyngeal airway may help to keep the airway open and more stable during bag-mask ventilation. Consider other airway management options.

2. *What airway techniques could be considered to manage this difficult airway?*

Continue bag-mask ventilation and check oxygenation on pulse oximetry. If the patient's oxygen saturation can be maintained around 90%, then transport.

If not, RSI could be problematic in this case as the intubation is difficult and the patient has suffered facial injuries that could distort airway anatomy. The patient is too young to use the gum elastic bougie to facilitate intubation. If an LMA is available, place it and reassess the patient. The LMA has been used to manage trauma patients with cervical spine immobilization. If LMA is not available and the airway cannot be maintained any other way, perform needle cricothyrotomy.

Quick Quiz

1. *The gum elastic bougie is used to facilitate intubation in which age group of patients?*
   A. Infants
   B. Children younger than 2 years of age
   C. Children younger than 12 years of age
   D. Adolescents 14 years or older and adults

2. *RSI is contraindicated in which of the following patients?*
   A. A 2-year-old girl in respiratory failure after a submersion injury (drowning).
   B. A 3-year-old boy in severe respiratory distress after choking on a superball.
   C. A 4-year-old asthmatic in respiratory failure.
   D. A 6-year-old boy with severe head trauma and a Glasgow Coma Scale score of 3 after being struck by a car.

3. *During RSI, children may be given atropine to prevent which of the following complications?*
   A. Aspiration
   B. Bradycardia
   C. Malignant hyperthermia
   D. Vomiting

4. *Potential advantages of the LMA over endotracheal intubation include which of the following?*
   A. Easier to learn the procedure.
   B. Procedure can be completed quickly.
   C. Avoids risk of esophageal intubation or mainstem bronchus intubation.
   D. All of the above.

5. *Which of the following statements describes why needle cricothyrotomy is rarely performed in the prehospital setting?*
   A. Complications are high.
   B. It requires the use of needles.
   C. It takes too long to perform the procedure.
   D. The cost of supplies is too great.

Glossary

arytenoids cartilages   Two small cartilages to which the vocal cords are attached and which are situated at the upper back part of the larynx.

carina   The point at which the trachea branches into the right and left mainstem bronchi.

cricothyroid membrane   A thin sheet of fascia that connects the thyroid and cricoid cartilages that make up the larynx.

fasciculations   Small local muscle contractions.

gum elastic bougie   A long stylet made of woven polyester and covered with resin.

hyperkalemia   High potassium levels.

hypoxemia   Low oxygen concentrations in blood cells.

laryngeal mask airway   A device that consists of a large bore tube with a distal inflatable molded mask placed above the laryngeal inlet to direct gases into the lungs.

left lateral decubitus position   A position in which the patient is on his or her left side.

malignant hyperthermia   A condition of unstable temperature and cardiovascular control.

mediastinum   The space in the chest between the lungs and other chest organs.

needle cricothyrotomy   A technique that involves the placement of a needle or catheter into the cricothyroid membrane to bypass the upper airway and instill oxygen into the trachea.

percutaneous   Through the skin.

rapid sequence intubation   A technique that facilitates success of intubation by using medication to sedate and paralyze the patient.

subcutaneous emphysema   The presence of air in the soft tissues, which creates a crackling sensation, called crepitus, felt on palpation.

succinylcholine   A drug used to facilitate intubation; produces muscle paralysis.

thyroid cartilage   The chief cartilage of the larynx; Adam's apple.

Selected References

1. Berry AM, Brimacombe JR, Verghase C. The laryngeal mask airway in emergency medicine, neonatal resuscitation, and intensive care medicine. *Int Anesthesiol Clin.* 1998;36:91–109.

2. Brimacombe JR, Berry A. The incidence of aspiration associated with the laryngeal mask airway: A meta-analysis of published literature. *J Clin Anesth.* 1995; 7:297–305.

3. Brownstein D, Shugerman R, Cummings P, et al. Prehospital endotracheal intubation of children by paramedics. *Ann Emerg Med.* 1996;28:1:34–39.

4. Idris AA, Gabriellai A. Advances in airway management. *Emerg Clin N Am.* 2002;20:843–857.

5. Le DH, Reed DB, Weinstein G, et al. Paramedic use of endotracheal tube introducers for the difficult airway. *Prehosp Emerg Care.* 2002;5:155–158.

6. www.LMANA.com, Accessed August 6, 2003.

7. McDonald CC, Bailey B. Out-of-hospital use of neuromuscular-blocking agents in the United States. *Prehosp Emerg Care.* 1998;2:29–32.

8. Mizelle HL, Rothrock SG, Silvestri S, Pagane J. Preventable morbidity and mortality from prehospital paralytic assisted intubation: Can we expect outcomes comparable to hospital-based practice. *Prehosp Emerg Care.* 2002;6:472–475.

9. Moscati R, Jehle D, Christiansen G, et al. Endotracheal tube introducer for failed intubations: A variant of the gum elastic bougie. *Ann Emerg Med.* 2000;36:52–56.

10. Nocera A. A flexible solution for emergency intubation difficulties. *Ann Emerg Med.* 1996;27:665–667.

11. Nolan JP, Wilson ME. Orotracheal intubation in patients with potential cervical spine injuries. An indication for the gum elastic bougie. *Anesthesia.* 1993;48:630–633.

12. Pennant JH, Walker MB. Comparison of the endotracheal tube and laryngeal mask in airway management by paramedical personnel. *Anesth Analg.* 1992;74:531–534.

13. Pitt K, Woollard M. Should paramedics bougie on down? *Pre-Hosp Immediate Care.* 2000;4:68–70. Available at http://www.asancep.org.uk/ShouldParamedicBougieonDown.htm. Accessed February 20, 2004.

14. Robinson KJ, Katz R, Jacobs LM. A 12-year experience with prehospital cricothyrotomies. *Air Med J.* 2002; 20:27–30.

15. Rumball CJ, MacDonald D. The PTL, Combitube, laryngeal mask, and oral airway: A randomized prehospital comparative study of ventilatory device effectiveness and cost-effectiveness in 470 cases of cardiorespiratory arrest. *Prehosp Emerg Care.* 1997;1:1–10.

16. Sasada MP, Gabbott DA. The role of laryngeal mask airway in pre-hospital care. *Resuscitation.* 1994;28:97–102.

17. Sing RF, Reilly PM, Rotondo MF, Lynch MJ, McCans JP, Schwab CW. Out-of-hospital rapid-sequence induction for intubation of the pediatric patient. *Acad Emerg Med.* 1997;4:80–81.

18. Spaite DW, Maralee J. Prehospital cricothyrotomy: An investigation of indications, technique, complications, and patient outcome. *Ann Emerg Med.* 1990;19:279–285.

19. Wayne MA, Friedland E. Prehospital use of succinylcholine: A 20-year review. *Prehosp Emerg Care.* 1999; 3:107–109.

Technology Resources

Online Course

Anatomy Review

Online Glossary

Web Links

Online Quiz

Scenarios

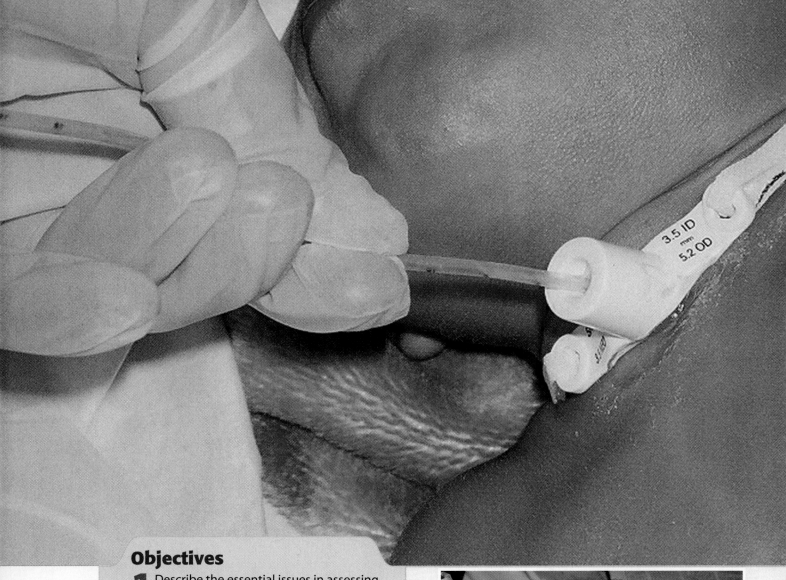

Objectives

1 Describe the essential issues in assessing and managing the airway of the patient with a tracheostomy.

2 Recognize the different types of tracheostomy tubes and their associated parts, accessories, and functions.

3 Identify the most common problems that result in the need for a tracheostomy in the pediatric patient, and the most common complications that can occur.

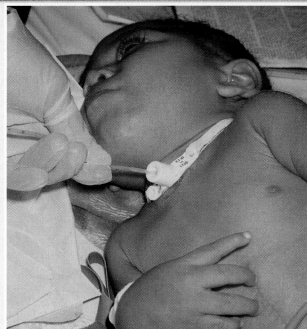

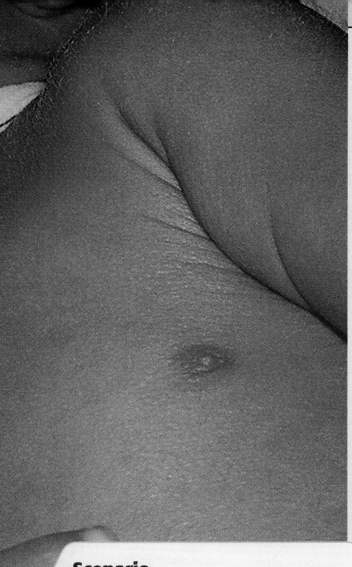

CHAPTER 9

Special Needs: Tracheostomy

Scenario

You respond to the home of a 3-year-old boy in respiratory distress where anxious parents inform you that he was recently discharged from the hospital with a tracheostomy tube in place. This morning the boy developed shortness of breath and increased work of breathing. He is intermittently awake but not responsive to you. His parents tell you that this has been normal behavior for him since he experienced a head injury several months ago.

1. *How do you assess the respiratory status of a patient with a tracheostomy?*

2. *What are the most important steps in the management of this patient?*

Think about these questions and this case as you read on. We will return to this scenario at the end of the chapter.

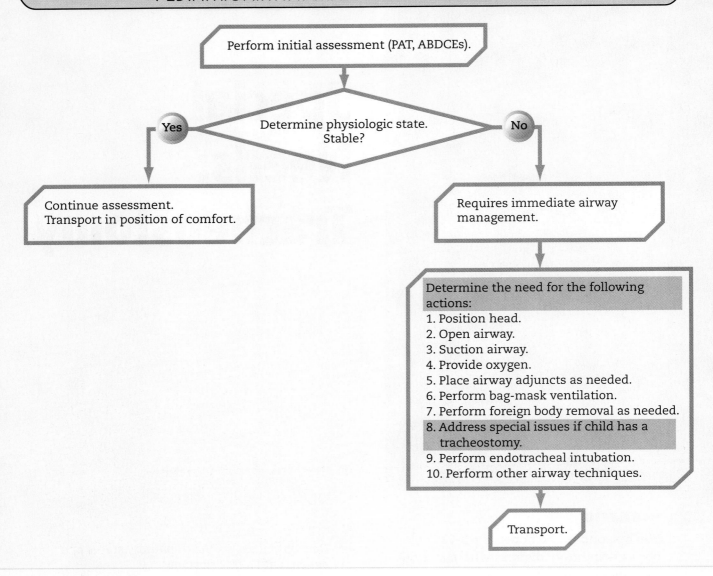

Perform initial assessment (PAT, ABDCEs).

Yes — Determine physiologic state. Stable? — **No**

Continue assessment.
Transport in position of comfort.

Requires immediate airway management.

Determine the need for the following actions:
1. Position head.
2. Open airway.
3. Suction airway.
4. Provide oxygen.
5. Place airway adjuncts as needed.
6. Perform bag-mask ventilation.
7. Perform foreign body removal as needed.
8. Address special issues if child has a tracheostomy.
9. Perform endotracheal intubation.
10. Perform other airway techniques.

Transport.

■ Introduction

The care of a patient with a tracheostomy poses some challenges and requires some specialized knowledge, but the basic principles of airway management are the same as for other patients. Airway management for these patients requires you to be familiar with the equipment, the names of each part of the equipment, how it functions, what purpose it serves, and the special anatomical considerations specific to a tracheostomy. With this knowledge, you will be prepared to assess and treat a child with special needs who has an airway emergency.

A tracheostomy is a surgical opening into the trachea or windpipe that allows passage of air for breathing (Figure 9–1).

The indications for initial tracheostomy placement are, for the most part: 1) upper airway obstruction due to congenital abnormalities, trauma, or surgery; 2) prolonged mechanical ventilation; and 3) impaired abil-

ity to clear airway secretions. The tracheostomy can be temporary or permanent. The stoma, or opening into the neck, is usually quite small, and requires a tracheostomy tube to keep it patent. The child breathes partially or completely through this tube.

A tracheostomy tube is a hollow tube made of metal or plastic, designed to fit into the surgical opening in the trachea to allow passage of air for breathing. The sizes of tracheostomy tubes range from 2.5 mm (neonates) to 10 mm (for adolescents or adults), although these sizes may vary slightly from one manufacturer to another. Tracheostomy tubes have a standard opening; they rarely need an adapter to connect to a bag-mask device for assisted ventilation. There are three types of tracheostomy tubes which vary in material composition, length, curvature, shape, and diameter:
1. *Single cannula tube.* Most pediatric tracheostomy tubes are of this type (Figure 9–2). Single cannula tubes are used for pediatric patients because of

Where's the Evidence?

Prehospital Care of Special Health Care Needs Patients

In a study by Spaite and colleagues, 2% of EMS responses were for children with special health care needs. Of these responses, 52% were related to the child's special health care needs and 48% were for complaints common to all children. Of the 924 children with special needs entered into the study, 18% required airway management.

Spaite and colleagues also evaluated the effect of specialized training for paramedics in issues related to children with special health care needs. Prior to the educational program, comfort levels for paramedics in caring for these children were significantly lower than the comfort levels in caring for children requiring pediatric advanced life support. Comfort levels were significantly higher for performance of standard pediatric skills versus specialized management skills.

Training improved comfort levels, but the comfort levels deteriorated significantly over time. This suggests that prehospital providers must review infrequently used skills and knowledge at regular intervals.

1. Spaite DW, Conroy C, Tibbitts M. Use of emergency medical services by children with special health care needs. *Prehosp Emerg Care*. 2000;4:19–23.

2. Spaite DW, Karriker KJ, Seng, M. Increasing paramedics' comfort and knowledge about children with special health care needs. *Am J Emerg Med*. 2000;18:747–752.

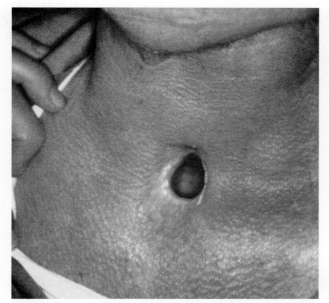

Figure 9–1 A tracheostomy is a surgical opening into the trachea or windpipe that allows passage of air for breathing.

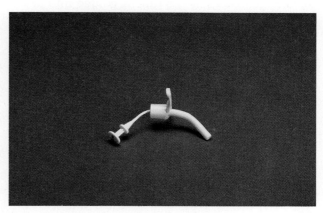

Figure 9–2 A single cannula tracheostomy tube.

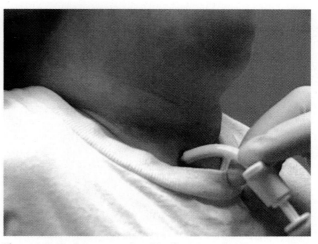

Figure 9–3 Tracheostomy tube with a flange or collar that rests against the neck.

the smaller diameter of the child's airway; when an inner cannula is added, the diameter of the airway becomes so small that it does not allow effective passage of air. Tracheostomy tubes have a flange or collar that rests against the neck once the tube is inserted. This prevents the tube from descending into the airway, and has slots for attaching tracheostomy ties to keep the tube in place (Figure 9–3).

2. *Double cannula tube.* This type of tracheostomy tube has an inner and an outer cannula. The

inner cannula must be in place to provide mechanical ventilation, and is removable for cleaning (Figure 9–4). Although the addition of the inner cannula facilitates cleaning of the tube, it also decreases the diameter of the already narrow opening increasing the likelihood of obstruction from secretions in small children. The inner cannula locks into place for security, and must be unlocked for removal.

3. *Fenestrated tube.* The third type of tracheostomy tube is a <u>fenestrated</u> (windowed) tube, which has an opening that allows air to pass up to the mouth and nose (Figure 9–4). This type of tracheostomy tube is used when the upper and lower airways are still connected; fenestration enables passage of air through the vocal cords so the patient can speak with the tracheostomy tube in place.

An <u>obturator</u> is used to facilitate insertion of a tracheostomy tube. The obturator is a small cylinder with a rounded tip designed to slide into the tracheostomy tube. With the obturator inserted, the tracheostomy tube becomes a solid, smooth object that is less likely to damage tissues as the tube is guided into place. Once the tracheostomy tube is in place, the obturator must be removed immediately because its presence occludes the tube (Figure 9–5).

Tracheostomy tubes may be cuffed or uncuffed. Because of the small diameter of the airway lumen below the cricoid ring in infants and toddlers, the tracheostomy tube forms a seal in these patients and a cuff is not needed. For the older child, however, a tracheostomy tube with an inflatable cuff is used to assure a tight seal for the airway, just as it is for an endotracheal tube. The cuff on these tubes consists of a balloon surrounding the tube which is inflated after insertion. There is also a pilot balloon similar to the pilot balloon on an ET tube to show whether the cuff is inflated or not.

The tracheostomy tube is held in place by tracheostomy ties, narrow strips of cloth similar to shoelaces. One end of the tie is secured to one side of the tracheostomy tube through the slot on the edge of the tracheostomy tube collar; the other end is brought around the back of the patient's neck, slipped through the slot on the opposite side of the tracheostomy tube collar and tied securely, preferably with a square knot. The ties must be tied tightly enough to hold the tube in place even when the patient coughs; they should be loose enough to allow your small finger between the knot on the tie and the patient's neck.

Anatomical Considerations

video There are anatomical differences in children that affect tracheostomy management, such as:

- Children have a smaller tracheal diameter and shorter distance between the tracheal rings. Because of the small diameter, the tube can more easily be occluded with dried secretions layering on the inner wall of the tube. Airway secretions are normally cleared by coughing, and by cilia (hair cells) within the airway passages which sweep secretions upward. There are no similar mechanisms for clearing of tracheostomy tubes.

Indications

Indications for airway intervention in a patient with a tracheostomy tube include the following:

- Inadequate ventilation or oxygenation
- Dislodgement of tracheostomy tube
- Obstruction of tracheostomy tube
- Bleeding from the tracheostomy tube

The most likely causes of respiratory distress for a patient with a tracheostomy tube in place are blockage of the tube by secretions and tube dislodgement. The DOPE mnemonic can be used to remember

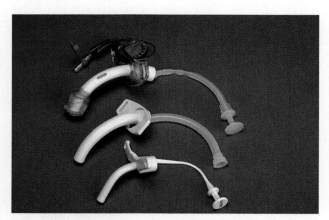

Figure 9–4 Fenestrated, double lumen, and single lumen tracheostomy tubes (top to bottom).

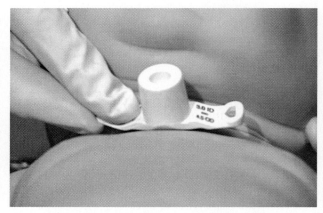

Figure 9–5 Remove the obturator from the tracheostomy once it has been inserted into the stoma.

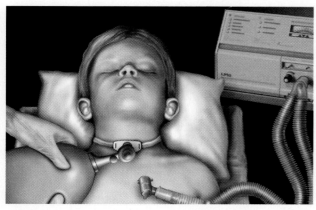

Figure 9–6 Remove the patient from the ventilator to eliminate this as the possible cause of the child's respiratory distress or failure, and begin bag-mask ventilation.

potential complications of tracheostomy. D – dislodgement; O – obstruction; P – pneumothorax; and E – equipment failure. If the patient is on a ventilator, remember to consider mechanical problems with the ventilator as another possible source of respiratory distress. Although less common, there may also be other medical problems such as asthma or anaphylaxis, or, rarely, obstruction by a foreign body.

In cases where your initial assessment shows that the child is having some difficulty breathing, but is not in acute respiratory distress, proceed with standard interventions such as suctioning and providing additional oxygen; you can then assess the patient for the cause of the distress.

If the patient is in acute respiratory distress or failure, additional intervention will be needed. When the patient is on a ventilator, the first step should be to remove the patient from the ventilator to eliminate this as a possible cause (Figure 9–6). For all patients in acute distress or failure, begin assisted ventilation with the bag-device (manual resuscitator) attached to the tracheostomy tube; this will allow you to perform your assessment, proceed with interventions, and attempt to determine the cause of the child's respiratory distress or failure.

Contraindications

Contraindications to airway intervention in a patient with a tracheostomy tube include:
- Patent airway with adequate chest rise

A patient with a tracheostomy tube who is in respiratory distress and has adequate chest rise may require only standard therapies such as suctioning, supplemental oxygen, or nebulized medications. Appropriate assessment and treatment for the cause of the respiratory distress is key to the management of these patients. Do not remove a tracheostomy tube

unless your assessment clearly shows the tracheostomy tube is obstructed and cannot be cleared by suctioning.

Procedure Step-by-Step

video The most likely causes of respiratory distress and/or failure in a patient with a tracheostomy tube are ventilator failure, obstruction of the tracheostomy tube, dislodgement of the tracheostomy tube, and bleeding or infection of the stoma.

Build-up of mucus in the tracheostomy tube is common, thus regular suctioning of the tracheostomy tube is necessary to remove these secretions from the tube and make it easier for the child to breathe. Parents and caregivers are usually trained in all aspects of tracheostomy care before the patient is discharged from the hospital, so they usually call for assistance when they are unable to solve the problem. Family members and caregivers are knowledgeable; use them as a resource, and do not be afraid to ask questions! They may have extra tubes, suction equipment including catheters, and supplies for cleaning the tube.

Tracheostomy Tube Obstruction
Assessment
Airway assessment of the patient with a tracheostomy tube is much the same as for any patient suspected of being in respiratory distress. Using the pediatric assessment triangle, check the airway, assess the work of breathing, and observe the child for circulatory status and level of consciousness. Signs of severe respiratory distress or failure include:
- Anxiety, restlessness, inconsolability, or altered level of consciousness
- Tachypnea
- Increased work of breathing (retractions, grunting, nasal flaring)
- Decreased breath sounds
- Abnormal skin signs (pale or cyanotic skin color, diaphoresis)
- Poor chest rise

Interventions for all patients with suspected tracheostomy tube obstruction include the following:
1. Position the head and neck for maximal airway opening.
2. If the patient is not breathing, or if there is inadequate chest rise with breathing, begin assisted ventilation with the bag-mask device (manual resuscitator) connected to the tracheostomy tube. Provide supplemental oxygen through the bag-mask device.
3. If attempts to assist ventilation through the tracheostomy tube are unsuccessful, attempt to clear the obstruction in the tracheostomy tube. When the patient has a single cannula

tube, this will involve instillation of saline followed by suctioning of the tracheal tube. If the patient has a double cannula, the inner cannula must be removed and cleaned to remove the obstruction. If these procedures fail, the tracheostomy tube will need to be removed and replaced.

4. Gather equipment and supplies. It is acceptable to ask the parents or home health care provider for suctioning apparatus and supplies, which should include: a functioning suction unit, suction tubing and sterile suction catheter of an appropriate size to fit down the tracheostomy tube, sterile saline, sterile water, 1–2 small sterile containers, and a trash bag for disposing of used supplies.

5. Wear appropriate personal protective equipment such as gloves, goggles, and a mask.

6. Maintain aseptic technique.

7. If possible, administer high-flow oxygen prior to beginning suctioning attempts.

Patients with Single Cannula Tracheostomy Tubes
Suctioning the Tracheostomy Tube
To suction a single cannula tracheostomy tube, perform the following steps:

1. Open a sterile suction catheter package and put a sterile glove on one hand. Pick up the suction catheter with that hand.

2. Holding the suction tubing with your other (non-sterile gloved) hand, connect the sterile catheter to the tubing without contaminating your sterile hand.

3. Swirl the tip of the sterile suction catheter in some sterile saline to make it easier to insert.

4. Turn on suction (to less than 100 mm Hg), but do not cover the suction control hole at this point.

5. Insert the catheter using the hand with the sterile glove until you meet resistance, approximately 2 to 3 inches. The catheter should follow the curve of the tracheostomy tube. Do not force the catheter past the point where you meet resistance, as it can cause trauma and bleeding to the airway and potentially cause a pneumothorax.

6. When the catheter is in far enough, place the thumb of your non-sterile hand over the suction control hole.

7. Slowly withdraw the suction tubing using a twisting or rotating motion as you withdraw it. Do not suction longer than 5 seconds.

8. Rinse the suction catheter by placing the tip of the catheter in the container of sterile saline and applying suction until the catheter is clear.

9. Allow the child to breathe several times between each suctioning attempt or provide assisted ventilation for a minimum of 30 to 60 seconds between attempts. Each time you suction, you are removing oxygen as well as secretions from the patient's lungs, so supply supplemental oxygen between attempts at suctioning.

10. Repeat the suctioning procedure until you feel you have effectively cleared the mucus and secretions from the tube and note improvements in the patient's signs, symptoms, and appearance.

Patients with Double Cannula Tracheostomy Tubes
Most pediatric tracheostomy tubes do not have inner cannulas, so you may be able to skip this step. If the tracheostomy tube has an inner cannula, the family should be able to provide you with necessary supplies including a pipe cleaner or tiny bottle brush suitable for cleaning it. Removal and cleaning of an inner cannula must be done rapidly when a patient requires assisted ventilation, as the bag ventilation device cannot be attached to the tracheostomy tube without the inner cannula in place. To remove and clean the inner cannula, perform the following steps:

1. "Unlock" the inner cannula by turning it counter-clockwise until the indicator is in the 12 o'clock position (i.e., under the chin).

2. Stabilize the outer cannula, hold it in place with one hand, and remove the inner cannula with the other hand.

3. Clean the inner cannula rapidly using sterile technique.

4. Determine that the obstruction is relieved in the inner cannula and then reinsert the inner cannula into the outer cannula. Stabilize the outer cannula with one hand while inserting the inner cannula with the other hand. When the inner cannula has been inserted completely, twist or turn the outer portion of the tube clockwise until it clicks, locking the inner cannula into place.

5. Perform bag-tracheostomy ventilation as needed.

Procedure Continued
Once suctioning has been performed and the inner cannula has been removed and cleaned (if applicable), perform the following steps. These steps apply to all patients regardless of the type of cannula he or she has.

1. Reassess the patient.
   a. Look for bilateral chest rise, listen for equal breath sounds, and observe the patient.
   b. Signs of continued obstruction include lack of chest rise, faint or absent breath

sounds, unusual resistance to assisted ventilation, and lack of improvement in patient status.

2. Dispose of contaminated supplies. Dispose of all used equipment, contaminated saline and water. The family may re-sterilize some of the equipment used, so confirm what is disposable before throwing anything away.

3. Consider possible causes for respiratory distress once the patient is being ventilated adequately. Remember that the cause may or may not be related to the patient's tracheostomy. Other causes of respiratory distress or failure in a patient with a tracheostomy are tracheostomy tube dislodgement, bleeding, infection, or rarely, pneumothorax.

Airway management of a patient with a tracheostomy tube is summarized in **Skill Drill 9–1**.

Tracheostomy Tube Replacement

When a tracheostomy tube has been removed because of obstructing secretions that could not be cleared, or if the tube has been dislodged, insert a new tube immediately to assure patency of the airway. Although inserting a replacement tube may be extremely difficult if the tracheostomy is less than one week old, these children are routinely hospitalized for at least one week and are not discharged from the hospital until the tracheostomy is replaceable. Most parents are taught how to replace their child's tracheostomy tube, but they may encounter some difficulty, or they may not have a replacement tube available. The procedure for tracheostomy tube removal and replacement is as follows:

1. Assess the patient using the pediatric assessment triangle.

2. Reposition the head and neck for maximal airway opening if the patient is not ventilating adequately and the tracheostomy tube is clear.

3. Reassess the patient's ventilatory status. If ventilation is still inadequate, obtain a new tube and obturator (single cannula tube) and prepare to remove and replace the tube.

4. Remove the old tube. The new tube must be inserted rapidly to prevent closing of the stoma.

5. Insert the obturator into the new tracheostomy tube (single cannula); insert the inner cannula into the outer cannula of a double cannula tube if it has been removed.

6. Lubricate the tube with water-soluble jelly before insertion.

7. Insert the tube quickly into the tracheostomy stoma.

8. Do not force the tube when inserting it,. If you meet resistance, you may not be in the trachea; forcing it may create a false passage.

9. Make sure the tracheostomy tube has been correctly placed, then remove the obturator (single cannula tracheostomy tube) immediately and assess for airway patency.

10. Begin assisted ventilation with the manual resuscitator bag attached to the end of the tracheostomy tube, carefully holding the tube in place.

11. Tie the tracheostomy tube in place, making sure it is loose enough so you can just place your small finger between the tie and the patient's skin.

12. Reassess the patient's ventilatory status. Consider other causes of respiratory distress or failure if ventilation is inadequate.

13. Assess for signs of improper placement, including unequal chest rise, unequal breath sounds, and difficulty ventilating the patient. Also check for bleeding in the tube, and signs of subcutaneous air, such as swelling of the neck or crepitus.

14. Transport immediately.

■ Problem Solving

If secretions in the tube are very thick or dry, loosen or thin them by instilling 2 mL of sterile normal saline into the tracheostomy tube using either a small syringe without a needle or a soft plastic prefilled normal saline ampule (aka "pillow" or "bullet"). Instilling the saline will probably make the child start coughing—this is normal. After instilling the sterile normal saline, you may begin suctioning immediately.

If you are unable to reinsert a tracheostomy tube, reposition the child's head and neck. If the tube will still not enter, try to insert the old tube (check for patency before reinsertion). If the old tube cannot be inserted, attempt to insert a small ET tube (use pediatric length-based resuscitation tape for appropriate size, or measure the inner diameter of the ET tube against the nail of the child's little fingernail). If you have severe difficulty inserting the ET tube, you can thread a suction catheter through the lumen of the ET tube and then insert the catheter into the stoma. Once the catheter is in place, slide the ET tube over the catheter into the stoma. Once the ET tube is in place, remove the suction catheter and begin assisted ventilation with the manual resuscitator attached to the end of the ET tube. Transport the patient to the hospital immediately, continuing your respiratory assessment en route.

If there is no ET tube or tracheostomy tube available, attempt bag-mask ventilation with the mask over the nose and mouth of the patient while occluding the open stoma with a gauze pad. If there is no chest rise, this means that there is no connection between the mouth and the trachea. You must then place a small mask over the stoma and attempt mask-stoma ventilation. Transport the patient immediately.

Management strategies for caring for tracheostomy emergencies are outlined in **Figure 9–7**.

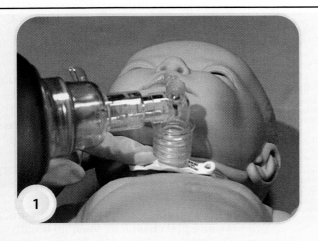

Position the patient. If the patient is on a mechanical ventilator, remove from ventilator and assist ventilation.

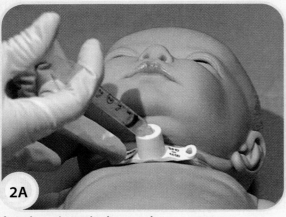
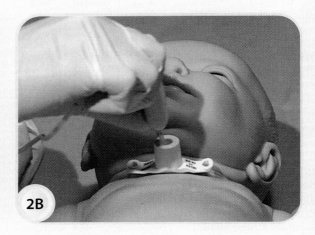

If no chest rise—single cannula:
- Instill 2 mL normal saline into the tracheostomy tube (**A**).
- Insert a sterile suction catheter through the tracheostomy tube until resistance is met (**B**).
- Suction for a maximum of 5 seconds, no higher than 100 mg Hg of pressure.

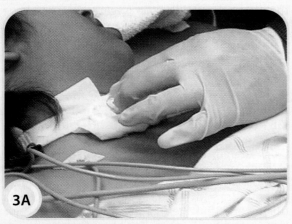
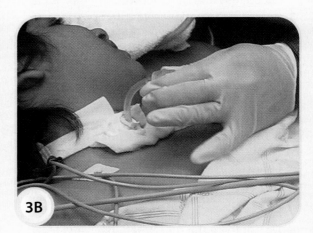

If no chest rise—double cannula:
- Remove the inner cannula (**A**).
- Clean the inner cannula (rapidly).
- Reinsert the inner cannula (**B**).

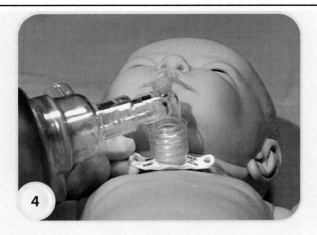

4

Place the manual resuscitation bag on the end of the tracheostomy tube and attempt to ventilate. Repeat the procedure.

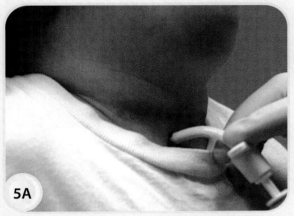

5A

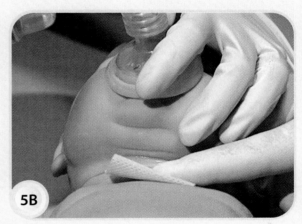

5B

If there is still no chest rise, remove the entire tracheostomy tube **(A)**.

- Begin bag-mask ventilation over the mouth and nose while your partner seals the stoma by holding a piece of gauze over the stoma with one hand **(B)**.

Do not pack gauze into the stoma.

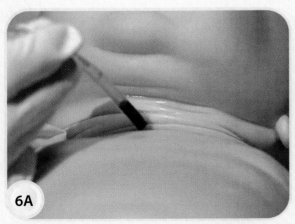

6A

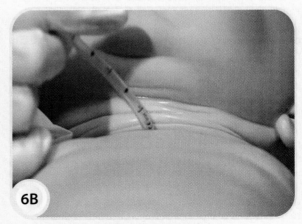

6B

If there is still no chest rise with bag-mask ventilation, replace the tracheostomy tube with a new tube.

- If no new tracheostomy tube is available, insert an appropriately sized ET tube into the tracheostomy stoma (ALS) **(A, B)**. ET tube size can be determined using one of the following methods:
  - A length-based pediatric resuscitation tape
  - Formula: $(Age/4) + 4$

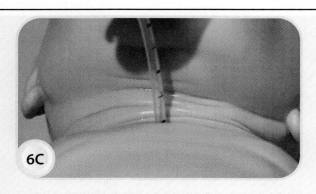

6C

- Insert the ET tube through the stoma approximately half the distance, as if the tube were inserted through the mouth **(C)**.

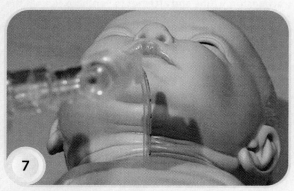

7

Attach the bag-mask device and attempt to ventilate. Assess for chest rise and fall.

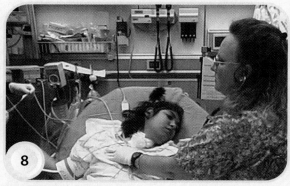

8

Repeat assessment.

Complications

Complications that can arise during airway intervention on a patient with a tracheostomy include the following:

- Trauma to tissues
- Formation of a false track during tracheostomy tube insertion. (If this is unrecognized and attempts are made to ventilate the patient through the false passage, subcutaneous emphysema with swelling of the neck and obstruction of the airway can occur rapidly.)
- Hypoxia
- Pneumothorax

Corrective Measures

Corrective measures to be taken when complications arise during airway intervention of a patient with a tracheostomy include the following:

- Tissue trauma: Be gentle, don't force tracheostomy tube or suction catheter past the point where resistance is met. Do not insert a tracheostomy tube without the obturator in place. Use no higher than 100 mg Hg of pressure when suctioning.
- When inserting a tracheostomy tube, stop inserting when resistance is met. Lubricate the tracheostomy tube and insert the obturator. Reassess patency of airway after insertion—

check for signs of subcutaneous emphysema or swelling of the neck.
- Count to 5 or have another provider check to make sure you do not suction for too long. Allow the child to take several breaths before making the next suction attempt.
- Be gentle with the suction catheter—do not force or insert the catheter too aggressively. Stop inserting as soon as you feel resistance. Once you meet resistance on insertion, withdraw the catheter slightly before applying suction to prevent damage to airway tissues.

TRICKS of the Trade

- Even if the child appears to be ventilating well, inadequate oxygenation may be evidenced by agitation, altered mental status, or change in skin color. Either situation should be considered a life-threatening emergency requiring critical intervention. If the patient appears seriously ill, immediate intervention will be necessary.

- An important question to ask as you begin supporting the child's ventilation is whether the child's upper airway is still connected to the lower airway. If you are unable to ventilate through the upper airway, ventilation through the stoma may be necessary.

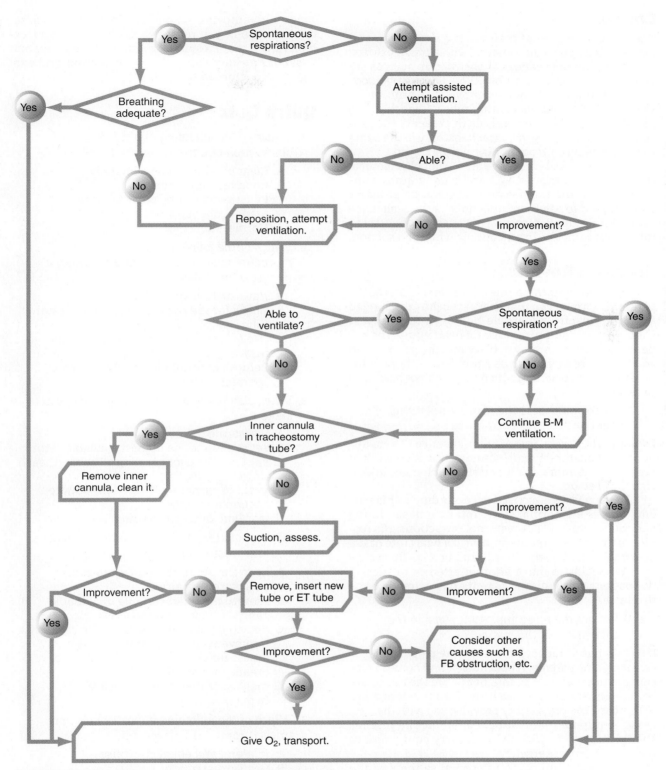

Figure 9–7 Algorithm for the management of tracheostomy emergencies.

Conclusions

The basic principles of maintaining ventilation and oxygenation apply when dealing with a tracheostomy. Assess for possible causes of obstruction such as secretions, mucus, swelling, bleeding, and foreign bodies. Suctioning can help remove the buildup of secretions in the tracheostomy tube. Other than the need to clean the inner cannula (if present), the procedure for suctioning via a tracheostomy is the same as the procedure for suctioning via an ET tube.

The family and caregivers are a valuable resource; they have been trained and are usually quite comfortable with the tracheostomy. Do not be afraid or embarrassed to ask them questions or for assistance in obtaining supplies, setting up a new tracheostomy tube, or cleaning the inner cannula while you suction.

Scenario Review

You responded to the home of a 3-year-old boy. His parents informed you that he was recently discharged from the hospital where he had been for the past 3 months after suffering a severe head injury. The patient has a tracheostomy in place and the parents told you that there seemed to be a problem with the tube, possibly an obstruction, which they had not been able to resolve.

1. *How do you assess the respiratory status of a patient with a tracheostomy tube?*

Look for chest rise, presence or absence of respirations, and bilateral breath sounds, increased work of breathing, alteration in mental status, changes in skin signs, and so on.

The boy is semi-conscious; according to his parents, this is his normal state. You note nasal flaring and intercostal and suprasternal retractions. His respiratory rate is 36 breaths/min with a heart rate of 120 beats/min. His fingernail beds and lips are dusky.

You decide to make another attempt to suction the patient although the parents have already done this once.

2. *What are the most important steps in the management of this patient?*

If a child has a tracheostomy, anyone responsible for care including parents, school nurses, and home health care providers should be taught to have the necessary equipment and how to use it should a problem arise. In this case, the boy's father provides you with the necessary equipment and supplies. All mobile rescues should be stocked with the necessary equipment to handle such an emergency.

After you instill 2 mL of normal saline into the child's single cannula tracheostomy tube, he starts coughing and expels a large mucous plug from the opening of the tracheostomy tube. You suction the tracheostomy tube, repeating the procedure two more times and removing a moderate amount of thick secretions. When you reassess, the boy no longer exhibits any signs of respiratory distress. Retractions and nasal flaring have stopped, color is normal, and vital signs have returned to normal.

Quick Quiz

1. *Which of the following might indicate obstruction of a tracheostomy tube?*

   A. Clear breath sounds bilaterally
   B. Good respiratory effort
   C. Bilateral wheezing on auscultation
   D. Inadequate chest rise
   E. Normal skin color

2. *Which of the following is not the correct procedure when removing and replacing a tracheostomy tube?*

   A. Have suction available.
   B. Check for the correct size of tracheostomy tube.
   C. Use force to overcome resistance on insertion.
   D. Remove obturator after tube insertion.
   E. Tie tracheostomy ties securely.

3. *When suctioning a tracheostomy tube, you should:*

   A. use sterile technique.
   B. set suction to the highest available setting.
   C. suction for no longer than 15 seconds each time.
   D. avoid oxygenating the patient between suction attempts.
   E. use 2 mL of water to soften secretions.

4. *When providing ventilation with a bag device to a tracheostomy tube, you should:*

   A. keep the obturator in place to assure patency of the airway.
   B. remove the inner cannula of a double cannula tracheostomy tube.
   C. detach the oxygen line from the bag device to prevent giving too much oxygen.
   D. assess for chest rise and the presence of breath sounds bilaterally.
   E. make sure the patient's neck is hyperextended.

5. *Which of the following indicates improper tracheostomy tube placement?*

   A. Bilateral and equal chest rise
   B. Gastric distention
   C. Swelling of the neck with crepitus
   D. Coughing
   E. Deposit of secretions inside the tracheostomy tube

Glossary

cannula   A tube for insertion into a vessel or other passageway such as the nasal passage.

crepitus   A grinding or crackling sensation felt upon palpation of the skin; can be due to the presence of air in the soft tissues (subcutaneous emphysema) or broken bone ends.

diaphoresis   Profuse sweating.

fenestrated   A type of tracheostomy tube that has an opening or window.

obturator   A small cylinder with a rounded tip designed to slide into the tracheostomy tube; with this inserted, the tracheostomy tube becomes a solid, smooth object that is less likely to damage tissues as the tube is guided into place.

stoma   An opening in the body, usually in the neck; when in the neck, its purpose is to connect the trachea directly to the skin for ventilation.

Selected References

1. American Heart Association, International Liaison Committee on Resuscitation. Guidelines 2000 for Cardiopulmonary Resuscitation and Emergency Cardiovascular Care: An International Consensus on Science. *Circulation*. 2000;102(suppl I):I-253–I-290.

2. American Heart Association, International Liaison Committee on Resuscitation. Guidelines 2000 for Cardiopulmonary Resuscitation and Emergency Cardiovascular Care: An International Consensus on Science. *Circulation*. 2000;102(suppl I):I-291–I-342.

3. Bahng SC, VanHala S, Nelson VS, Hurvitz EA. Parental report of pediatric tracheostomy care. *Arch Phys Med Rehabil*. 1998;79:11:1367–1369.

4. Bosch JD, Cuyler JP. Home care of the pediatric tracheostomy: our experience. *J Otolaryngol*. 1987;16:2:120–122.

5. Dieckmann RA, Brownstein D, Gausche-Hill M (eds). *Pediatric Education for Prehospital Professionals: PEPP Textbook*. Sudbury, Mass: Jones and Bartlett Publishers; 2000.

6. Dorsey L, Diehl B. An educational program for school nurses caring for the pediatric client with tracheostomy: Training the school nurse to care for a child re-entering the public education system with a tracheostomy. *Ostomy Wound Management*. 1992;38:5:16–19.

7. Duncan BW, Howell LJ, deLorimier AA, et al. Tracheostomy in children with emphasis on home care. *J Pediatr Surg*. 1992;27:4:432–435.

8. Foltin G, Tunik M, Cooper D. (eds.) et al. *Paramedic Teaching Resource for Instructors in Prehospital Pediatrics (TRIPP)*. New York: Center for Pediatric Emergency Medicine: 2001. http://www.cpem.org/html/trippals.html. Accessed February 27, 2004.

9. Gaudet PT, Peerless A, Sasaki CT, Kirchner JA. Pediatric tracheostomy and associated complications. *Laryngoscope*. 1978;88:10:1633–1641.

10. Gausche M, Goodrich SM, Poore PD. *Instructor Manual for Advanced Life Support Providers: Pediatric Airway Management Project*; 2nd ed. Torrance, CA: Maternal and Child Health Bureau. National Highway Traffic and Safety Administration and the Agency for Healthcare Research and Quality, 1997. Includes full slide set.

11. Lichtenstein MA. Pediatric home tracheostomy care: a parent's guide. *Pediatr Nursing*. 1986;12:1: 41–48, 69.

12. Mullins JB, Templer JW, Kong J, et al. Airway resistance and work of breathing in tracheostomy tubes. *Laryngoscope*. 1993;103:12:1367–1372.

13. Hazinsky MF, Zaritsky AL, Nadkarni VM (eds.), et al. *PALS Provider Manual*. Dallas, Texas: American Heart Association; 2002.

14. Peirson GS. Home care protocols for pediatric tracheostomy patients. *Caring*. 1993;2:12:38–42.

15. Shaw A. Caring for the child with a tracheostomy. *J Pract Nurs*. 1975;25:10:28–30.

16. Simma B, Spehler D, Burger R, et al. Tracheostomy in Children. *Eur J Pediatr*. 1994;153:4:291–296.

17. Spaite DW, Conroy C, Tibbitts M, et al. Use of emergency medical services by children with special health care needs. *Prehosp Emerg Care*. 2000;4:19–23.

18. Sullivan MJ, Hom DB, Passamani PP, DiPietro MA. An unusual complication of tracheostomy. *Archives of Otolaryngol Head Neck Surgery*. 1987;113:2: 198–199.

19. Warnock C, Porpora K. A pediatric tracheostomy card: transforming research into practice. *Pediat Nursing*. 1994;20:2:186–188.

End of Chapter Activities

Technology Resources

Online Course

Anatomy Review

Online Glossary

Web Links

Online Quiz

Scenarios

Quick Quiz Answers

Chapter 1: Introduction

1. **A.** Children represent 10% of prehospital calls; of these, 5% are life- or limb- threatening.

2. **A.** The epiglottis is floppy and U-shaped, the occiput is prominent, and the cricoid is the narrowest portion of the airway. Other differences are that (i) the tongue is relatively large; (ii) the trachea is shorter; (iii) the trachea rings are more flexible; (iv) the vocal cords are c-shaped; and (v) children have a faster metabolic rate and less well developed chest and abdominal musculature.

3. **C.** Suctioning the nose to remove secretions will allow for a clear airway passage. Placing a towel under the shoulders is a proper maneuver for head positioning but will not relieve airway obstruction in the nose. Placing a nasopharyngeal airway is not recommended in infants younger than 1 year of age. In addition, the small diameter of pediatric nasal airways allows them to easily become occluded with mucous. A nasal cannula may be used in infants but provides very little supplemental oxygen and cannot relieve obstruction of the nose from secretions.

4. **D.** You can participate in improving EMSC by advocating for changes in education and training, prevention programs, patient care protocols, system policies, and legislation at federal, state, and local levels. Individually, you can prepare your station or service for a critical child emergency by ensuring that you have the appropriate size equipment and supplies available; obtaining the knowledge of pediatric emergency care necessary to assess and treat an infant, child, or adolescent; and practicing pediatric airway management skills to maintain a high level of proficiency in the care of critically ill or injured pediatric patients.

5. **D.** Respiratory distress is defined as a condition characterized by increased work of breathing as a result of tissue hypoxia. Poor tidal volume and cyanosis may be present in both respiratory failure and respiratory distress but neither condition defines respiratory distress. Prolonged absence of breathing is respiratory arrest.

Chapter 2: Assessment

1. **E.** The Pediatric Assessment Triangle consists of assessment of the child's appearance, work of breathing, and circulatory status. Level of consciousness is assessed as one part of the child's appearance; interactivity is also an important component.

2. **A.** Vital signs, especially blood pressure, are less reliable in assessing the pediatric patient than the level of alertness and interactivity. Yet assessing vital signs remains an important part of the assessment of all patients.

3. **E.** Increased respiratory rate with increased work of breathing indicates respiratory distress. Children can increase their respiratory rates dramatically in response to hypoxia, and because of their less well developed musculature, they show retractions more readily than adults. Recognition of these symptoms is key to early identification of respiratory distress.

4. **D.** Retractions are caused by increased work of breathing, a good indicator of respiratory distress.

5. **D.** Stridor is caused by obstruction of the passage of air through upper airway structures; it is an abnormal upper airway sound. Rales (crackles) may indicate disease of the lungs and can be seen with lower airway obstruction. Wheezing is also an abnormal lower airway sound and indicates lower airway obstruction. Rhonchi are low-pitched sounds caused by partial obstruction of the airway.

Chapter 3: Managing the Pediatric Airway in a Step-by-Step Approach

1. **A.** Begin with positioning the head, suctioning, and providing supplemental oxygen. Your next priority will be to stop the seizure. Endotracheal intubation should NOT be attempted. Reassess the need for support of ventilation.

2. **A.** This patient is in cardiopulmonary arrest and requires support of ventilation and oxygen as soon as possible. The simplest way to provide these is by the management steps listed in A. These steps should be followed by chest compressions and assessment of cardiac rhythm. Further management priorities will be guided by these interventions and assessments. Endotracheal intubation may follow depending on a number of factors such as response to bag-mask ventilations, proximity to the emergency department, and skill of the provider. Foreign body aspiration is unlikely in this age group but should be considered if there is no chest rise with bag-mask ventilation.

3. **D.** The first step is to open the airway and if the foreign body is visible remove it, and perform bag-mask ventilation. If there is no chest rise, try abdominal thrusts to dislodge the foreign body. Check the mouth again for a foreign body and if one is not visible, perform bag-mask ventilation again. If there is no chest rise, then perform laryngoscopy and remove the foreign body if visualized. After the foreign body is removed, perform bag-mask ventilation. Advanced maneuvers such as endotracheal intubation around the foreign body or cricothyrotomy may result in worsening the patient's condition and could be considered only after these initial maneuvers fail.

4. **B.** Pediatric airway management includes assessment of need followed by the performance of a graduated series of skills based on that assessment followed by reassessment of the success of those skills in improving the patient's condition. Although you may be performing skills that you do not use regularly, you may have to use them if your assessment of the child determines that the skill is necessary to support oxygenation or ventilation. This is why continuing education and skill practice is vital. Some skills may be associated with higher risk and should be performed if you assess that the benefit of the procedure outweighs its risk to the patient.

Chapter 4: Positioning the Patient and Opening the Airway

1. **C.** To open the airway in an infant and young child, keep the head in the midline and neutral position, and place a small towel under the shoulders.

2. **D.** Nasopharyngeal airways are used in patients who are semiconscious or may return to consciousness, as in a seizing patient. All of the other answers listed are contraindications or relative contraindications.

3. **A.** An improperly sized oropharyngeal airway can push the tongue into the posterior pharynx, ob-

structing the airway. The oropharyngeal airway would not be long enough to enter the esophagus nor likely to cause lacerations of the tongue unless it is cut. Trimming any airway adjunct can lead to sharp edges and lacerations and should not be done.

4. **C.** When placing a nasopharyngeal airway in the right nostril there is no need to rotate it as the curve of the nasopharyngeal airway follows the anatomic curve of the patient's nasopharynx. The nasopharyngeal airway should be lubricated prior to insertion to avoid friction trauma in the nose (bleeding) and the bevel of the airway should always be facing the septum upon insertion.

Chapter 5: Bag-Mask Ventilation

1. **C.** Size the mask from the bridge of the nose to the cleft of the chin. This avoids compression of the eyes and allows for the best seal of the mask over the nose and the mouth.

2. **C.** The patient's lower chest begins to rise. Once this chest rise is initiated, release the bag to allow for exhalation. In infants and young children, the lower chest and upper abdomen will go up and down with the ventilation cycle. This is normal. A mid and upper abdomen that continues to expand in size denotes that air is going into the esophagus and inflating the stomach.

3. **A.** Pressure on the submental area (under the chin) can lead to upper airway obstruction in two ways: i) by direct compression of airway structures or ii) by pushing the tongue into the posterior pharynx (back of the mouth). Airway injury would occur only if intentional and excessive force were used.

4. **B.** Delivering breaths with slower inspiration times and with adequate volumes allows for air to go into the trachea and lungs but not too much air to enter the esophagus. As increased pressure is used the esophagus opens and air fills the stomach. If too much volume is delivered, then the lungs fill rapidly but excessive air fills the stomach. Eventually too much air in the stomach will prevent the diaphragm from its normal movement which can lead to hypoventilation.

Chapter 6: Foreign Body Removal

1. **C.** Vocal sounds are made with the passage of air through airway structures. Inability to speak or make sounds suggests complete airway obstruction.

2. **C.** When an object is below the vocal cords, it is not only difficult to reach, but you risk worsening the obstruction and damaging airway structures by attempting to remove it.
3. **A.** It would be difficult to convert a partial obstruction to a complete obstruction when only BLS procedures are used. Improper use of a laryngoscope and Magill forceps can potentially push the foreign body further into the airway and result in complete obstruction.
4. **B.** The statement is FALSE. Blind finger sweeps are not used at any point in airway management of children. There is risk of worsening the airway obstruction by pushing the object further into the posterior pharynx or trachea. If an object is visualized in the mouth, it can be removed, but blind finger sweeps are not appropriate.

Chapter 7: Endotracheal Intubation

1. **C.** When oxygen is inhaled into the lungs in normal respiration, gas exchange occurs, resulting in exhalation of carbon dioxide. Carbon dioxide can be detected by the use of a device attached to an endotracheal tube. If carbon dioxide is not detected by this device, the tube may be in the esophagus (esophageal intubation); this would result in death of the patient if the tube is not removed. The colorimetric detector assists in determining the location of the endotracheal tube—whether it is mistakenly inserted into the esophagus or correctly inserted into the trachea. The esophageal detector device is a suction device which relies on the difference in pliability of the trachea vs. the esophagus to determine tube placement. The Sellick maneuver involves using cricoid pressure during intubation. Auscultation of breath sounds bilaterally may assist in determining correct placement of the endotracheal tube, but does not bear any relation to carbon dioxide measurement.
2. **C.** The best indicator of correct endotracheal tube placement is visualizing the tube going past the vocal cords. Once past the vocal cords, the tube should not be advanced any further. When breath sounds are heard only on the right side of the chest, it is likely that the mainstem bronchus is intubated, and the tube should be withdrawn until breath sounds are heard bilaterally. Because of the differences in individual anatomy, the length that the tube must be inserted will vary from person to person. This can be estimated by multiplying the tube size by 3 corresponding to the cm markings on the side of the tube.
3. **A.** One possible benefit of endotracheal intubation is that it provides a pathway for administration of medications when an intravenous or intraosseous line is not available. The benefits of this, however, must be very carefully weighed against the possible complications, including airway trauma, esophageal intubation, and tube dislodgement, among others. The skills required for use of pediatric endotracheal intubation have been shown to deteriorate rapidly, so practice and skill maintenance are essential if this skill is to be included as an option for airway management.
4. **B.** The Sellick maneuver involves application of cricoid pressure, which can assist in closing the patient's esophagus; this may prevent gastric insufflation as well as aspiration of gastric contents. The Sellick maneuver may also help in visualizing the vocal cords, but it does not prevent right mainstem bronchus intubation, nor does it assist in detecting esophageal intubation.

Chapter 8: Advanced Techniques in Pediatric Airway Management

1. **D.** The elastic gum bougie is used in adolescents age 14 years or older and adults. In younger children, the softer tracheal rings may limit its use.
2. **B.** Upper airway obstruction is a contraindication to RSI as is abnormal airway anatomy (i.e., major facial trauma) and laryngeal fracture. In each of these cases, an alternative form of airway management will be necessary.
3. **B.** Atropine is given to prevent bradycardia that may occur with stimulation of the back of the throat or as a side effect of succinylcholine.
4. **D.** Studies of paramedical personnel's ability to perform LMA versus endotracheal intubation show that LMA can be taught more quickly (minutes); that the procedure can be performed faster (30 seconds versus over 100 seconds); and that complications such as esophageal intubation and mainstem bronchus intubation are avoided with the LMA.
5. **A.** The reason cricothyrotomy is rarely performed in the out-of-hospital setting is that complications are high: up to 40%. The cost of the materials is not high and the procedure can be performed quickly. The procedure requires the use of needles and a catheter, but needles are also used to place intravenous lines.

Chapter 9: Special Needs: Tracheostomy

1. **D.** Inadequate chest rise with good respiratory effort or severe retractions would be an indication that the tracheostomy tube is dislodged or displaced. When checking for tracheostomy tube ob-

struction, listen for clear and equal breath sounds bilaterally, observe chest for good respiratory effort, and check for normal skin color. Wheezing is not a sign of tracheostomy tube obstruction, although it may be a sign of asthma or anaphylaxis which can cause respiratory distress.

2. **C.** Using force to overcome resistance when inserting a tracheostomy tube can create a false channel and result in obstruction and subcutaneous emphysema. It is essential during this procedure to have suction available, check for the correct size of tracheostomy tube, and tie the tracheostomy ties securely. Removal of the obturator after tube insertion is necessary, as the obturator prevents passage of air through the tracheostomy tube.

3. **A.** Because the airway is vulnerable to infection, sterile technique should be used when suctioning a patient. A high setting on the suction device can damage the airway, and suctioning for over 5 seconds can result in inadequate oxygenation. It is important to oxygenate a patient either by manual resuscitator or by allowing the patient to breathe several times between suction attempts. Normal saline is used to soften secretions be-

cause it is isotonic and will cause less irritation to the airway than pure water.

4. **D.** Whenever you manage a patient's airway, you should assess for chest rise and presence of bilateral breath sounds at frequent intervals, along with circulatory assessment. The obturator of a single cannula tracheostomy tube must be removed, and the inner cannula of a double cannula tracheostomy tube must be in place when a manual resuscitator is used. Hyperextending a patient's neck may result in airway obstruction. Children should be placed in the sniffing position for maximal airway opening.

5. **C.** Swelling of the neck may indicate subcutaneous emphysema, a dangerous complication of improper tracheostomy tube placement. Bilateral and equal chest rise is a good sign that your airway management is effective. Gastric distention may be a complication of the use of a bag device with assisted ventilation, but does not indicate improper placement of the tracheostomy tube. Coughing and deposit of secretions inside the tracheostomy tube are common occurrences with tracheostomies, and are not necessarily signs of improper tube placement.

Glossary

A

accessory muscles　Muscles that assist in respiration.

acrocyanosis　Cyanosis of the extremities; this may be normal in the hands and feet of an infant within the first hour after birth.

adenoidal tissue　Lymphoid tissue in the back of the mouth and oropharynx.

airway adjunct　An artificial device to maintain an open airway.

alveoli　The air sacs of the lungs in which the exchange of oxygen and carbon dioxide takes place.

aphonia　Voice loss.

arytenoids cartilages　Two small cartilages to which the vocal cords are attached and which are situated at the upper back part of the larynx.

aspiration　The process of sucking in. Foreign bodies may be aspirated into the nose, throat, or lungs on inspiration.

auscultate　To listen to sounds within the body, usually with a stethoscope.

axilla　(plural = axillae) The armpit.

B

barotrauma　An injury caused by a change in pressure.

botulism　Food poisoning from consuming the bacterium *Clostridium botulinum* from spoiled food; illness is characterized by motor problems, visual problems, and dryness (for example, of airway).

bradycardia　A slow heartbeat.

bronchi　The two main branches leading from the trachea to the lungs, providing the passageway for air movement.

bronchioles　The smaller air passages in the lungs that extend from the bronchi to the alveoli.

C

cannula　A tube for insertion into a vessel or other passageway such as the nasal passage.

capnograph　A device used to confirm placement of an endotracheal tube; also called an end-tidal CO_2 detector.

cardiopulmonary arrest　A state in which no respiration and circulation are occurring; the patient is apneic and pulseless on examination.

cardiopulmonary failure　A state of inadequate respiration and circulation during which there is no breathing and no pulse.

carina　The point at which the trachea branches into the right and left mainstem bronchi.

colorimetric CO_2 detector　An instrument that determines the amount of carbon dioxide in expired air; measurements are represented by colors.

crackles　A series of short nonmusical sounds heard during inspiration, also called rales.

crepitus　A grinding or crackling sensation felt upon palpation of the skin; can be due to the presence of air in the soft tissues (subcutaneous emphysema) or broken bone ends.

cribriform plate　Perforated structure separating the nasal airway passage from the brain.

cricoid cartilage　The lowermost cartilage of the larynx.

cricoid pressure　The technique of placing pressure on either side of the cricoid cartilage on the neck to prevent gastric insufflation during endotracheal intubation; also called the Sellick maneuver.

cricoid ring　A ring of cartilage that encircles the larynx.

cricothyroid membrane　A thin sheet of fascia that connects the thyroid and cricoid cartilages that make up the larynx.

cyanosis　Slightly bluish, grayish, slatelike, or dark purple discoloration of the skin due to the presence of hypoxia.

D

decompensated shock　Shock associated with low blood pressure as compensatory mechanisms fail.

diaphoresis　Profuse sweating.

disease of the lungs　A condition that prevents adequate gas-exchange in the lung; this may be caused by the presence of fluid (edema or pus) or collapse or destruction of the air sacs (alveoli).

E

EC-clamp   A maneuver used to create an effective seal when ventilating a patient. An "E" is formed by placing the long, ring, and small fingers along the angle of the jaw. A "C" is formed by placing the thumb and index finger around the edge of the mask.

epigastrium   The abdominal area below the sternum.

epiglottis   A thin, leaf-shaped structure located immediately posterior to the root of the tongue that prevents food and secretions from entering the trachea.

epistaxis   Bleeding from the nose.

F

fasciculations   Small local muscle contractions.

fenestrated   A type of tracheostomy tube that has an opening or window.

G

gastric insufflation   The introduction of air into the stomach, which can be a complication of assisted ventilation; also called distention.

gum elastic bougie   A long stylet made of woven polyester and covered with resin.

H

hard palate   The hard portion of the roof of the mouth, separating the mouth from the nasal cavity.

head tilt-chin lift   A maneuver used to open the airway of a medical patient; in this maneuver, the forehead is tilted back and the chin is simultaneously lifted.

hyperkalemia   High potassium levels.

hypoventilation   A reduction in the normal amount of air that is entering the lungs, either from reduced rate and/or depth of breathing.

hypoxemia   Low oxygen concentrations in blood cells.

hypoxemic   Characterized by having deficient oxygenation in the blood.

hypoxia   Inadequate oxygen.

I

intercostal   Between the ribs.

J

jaw-thrust maneuver   A maneuver that can be used to open the airway of a trauma or medical patient; in this maneuver, two fingers are placed behind the angle of the jaw and the jaw is brought forward.

L

laryngeal mask airway   A device that consists of a large bore tube with a distal inflatable molded mask placed above the laryngeal inlet to direct gases into the lungs.

laryngoscopy   An examination of the interior of the larynx, usually done with a laryngoscope.

laryngospasm   A spasm of the laryngeal muscles.

larynx   The enlarged upper end of the trachea, below the root of the tongue, that contains the vocal cords.

left lateral decubitus position   A position in which the patient is on his or her left side.

lower airway obstruction   Obstruction of airflow from the mainstem bronchi to the end of the smallest air passages (bronchioles).

M

mainstem bronchus   Either of the two primary divisions of the trachea that lead respectively to the right and left lung.

malignant hyperthermia   A condition of unstable temperature and cardiovascular control.

manual resuscitator   A type of ventilation bag. There are two types: a self-inflating bag and an anesthesia bag. In the field, the self-inflating bag is also called a bag-mask device.

meconium   The thick, sticky, dark green first stools of the newborn.

mediastinum   The space in the chest between the lungs and other chest organs.

muscular dystrophy   An inherited condition involving weakness and atrophy of the muscles.

N

nasopharynx   The part of the pharynx situated above the soft palate and behind the nose.

needle cricothyrotomy   A technique that involves the placement of a needle or catheter into the cricothyroid membrane to bypass the upper airway and instill oxygen into the trachea.

O

obturator   A small cylinder with a rounded tip designed to slide into the tracheostomy tube; with this inserted, the tracheostomy tube becomes a solid, smooth object that is less likely to damage tissues as the tube is guided into place.

occiput   The back part of the skull.

oropharynx   The area of the pharynx located between the soft palate and upper part of the epiglottis.

P

palate The horizontal structure separating the mouth and the nasal cavity; the roof of the mouth.

partial nonrebreather mask A mask that adds a reservoir bag to increase inspired oxygen to 60%.

patency The state of being freely open.

patent Open and unobstructed.

Pediatric Assessment Triangle An assessment tool for obtaining an immediate general impression of the seriousness of an illness or injury by focusing on visual and auditory clues about appearance, work of breathing, and circulatory status of the infant or child.

percutaneous Through the skin.

pharynx Passageway for air (from nasal cavity to larynx) and food (from mouth to esophagus).

physiologic status State of a person's body functioning.

postictal A state after a seizure, in which the patient is confused.

pulse oximetry The measurement of oxygen saturation in the blood through the use of infrared technology; the device is clipped over the end of a finger or toe and oxygen saturation levels are displayed on a digital monitor.

R

rales A series of short nonmusical sounds heard during inspiration; also called crackles.

rapid sequence intubation A technique that facilitates success of intubation by using medication to sedate and paralyze the patient.

respiratory arrest A condition defined by absence of spontaneous respiration.

respiratory distress A condition characterized by increased work of breathing.

respiratory failure A condition where compensatory mechanisms are no longer able to maintain adequate oxygenation or ventilation.

retractions Physical drawing in of the chest wall between the ribs that occurs with increased work of breathing.

rhonchi A dry, low-pitched, snoring sound caused by partial obstruction of the airway.

S

Sellick maneuver The technique of placing pressure on either side of the cricoid cartilage on the neck to prevent gastric insufflation during endotracheal intubation; also called cricoid pressure.

stoma An opening in the body, usually in the neck; when in the neck, its purpose is to connect the trachea directly to the skin for ventilation.

stridor A harsh sound during inspiration, high-pitched due to partial upper airway obstruction.

subcutaneous emphysema The presence of air in the soft tissues, which creates a crackling sensation, called crepitus, felt on palpation.

submental area The area beneath the chin.

substernal Situated beneath the sternum.

succinylcholine A drug used to facilitate intubation; produces muscle paralysis.

supraclavicular Located above the clavicle.

T

thyroid cartilage The chief cartilage of the larynx; Adam's apple.

trachea A cylindrical cartilaginous tube from the larynx to the bronchial tubes. It extends from the 6th cervical to the 5th dorsal vertebra, where it divides at a point called the carina into two bronchi, one leading to each lung.

tragus Cartilaginous projection in front of the exterior meatus of the ear.

U

upper airway obstruction Obstruction of airflow from the level of the oropharynx to the mainstem bronchi.

V

vagal Pertaining to the vagus nerve and cholinergic nervous system.

vallecula The space between the base of the tongue and the epiglottis.

vocal cords Either of two pairs of folds of mucous membrane of which each member contains a band of fibrous tissue and a free edge projecting into the larynx.

W

wheezing Production of whistling sounds during expiration such as occurs in asthma and bronchiolitis.

X

xiphoid process The sword-shaped piece of cartilage located at the lower end of the sternum.

Index

Page numbers in *italics* designate figures, tables, and skill drills.

placement. *See* Oropharynx
size, 3, 5, 45, 58, 81
Trachea
  adults, contrast, 7
  damage, 100
  definition, 11
  endotracheal tube, location, *87*
  pressure, 70
  wire, insertion, *113*
Tracheal diameter, narrowness, 7, 69
Tracheal length, shortness, 5, 7
Tracheal opening, 45
Tracheal placement, confirmation. *See*
    Endotracheal tube
Tracheal rings
  compressibility, 69
  elasticity, 80
  stiffness, 99–100
Tracheal tube
  end-tidal CO$_2$ detector placement,
    38
  introducer, paramedic didactic
    session, 99
  suctioning, 122
Tracheostomy, 117. *See also* Permanent
    tracheostomy
  anatomical considerations, 120
  complications, 126
  contraindications, 121
  corrective measures, 126
  curve, 122
  emergencies, management
    algorithm, 127
  indications, 120–121
  obstruction, assessment, 121–122
  obturator, removal, 120
  pediatric airway management
    algorithm, 118
  problem solving, 123
  procedure, 121–123
  stoma, tube insertion, 123, 125
  surgical opening, illustration, 119
Tracheostomy tube, 118. *See also* Double
    lumen tracheostomy tubes;
    Fenestrated tracheostomy
    tubes; Single lumen
    tracheostomy tubes
  flange/collar, 119
  impact. *See* Bleeding
  improper placement, 128

obstruction, 120
  indication, 128
  procedure, 124–126
  replacement, 123
  suctioning, 128
  usage. *See* Double cannula
    tracheostomy tubes; Single
    cannula tracheostomy tubes
Traction, exertion, *90*
Tragus
  definition, 54
  measurement. *See* Nose
Trauma, 118
Trauma patients
  jaw-thrust maneuver, 50, 51
  positioning, 46–47
Tripod position. *See* Airway
TRIPP. *See* Teaching Resource for
    Instructors in Prehospital
    Pediatrics
Two-rescuer technique, usage, 61, 63

U

Unconscious child
  BLS maneuvers, indications, 70
  complete obstruction, procedure,
    72–73
Unconscious infant (0-1 yr.), 39
  complete obstruction, procedure, 71
Unconscious patient, airway adjunct
    (usage), 46
Uncuffed tubes, usage, 6
Unresponsive. *See* Alert Verbal Pain
    Unresponsive
  child, 54
Upper airway bypass, 111
Upper airway obstruction, 16, 111
  definition, 9, 11
  signs, 28
Upper airway trauma, 36
Upside-down rotation method, usage,
    51

V

Vagal
  definition, 54
  stimulation, 53

Vallecula, 81
  definition, 94
  laryngoscope blade, placement, 84
Ventilation, 112, *113*. *See also* Bag-
    mask ventilation
  adequacy, 82
    assessment, 36
  attempt, 71–73, *72, 126*
  inadequacy, 120
  initiation, 110
  performing. *See* Rescue ventilation
  providing, 128
  rates, slowing, 61
  requirement. *See* Assisted
    ventilation
  support, 38–39
  usage, 38
Ventilator, removal, 121
Verbal stimuli. *See* Alert Verbal Pain
    Unresponsive
Vital signs, 23–24
Vocal cords
  definition, 11
  endotracheal tube advancement, 85
  gum elastic bougie (flexed end),
    insertion, 100
  hiding, 81
  trauma, 36
  visualization, 74, *99*
    difficulty, 5
Vomiting, 46
  complications, 36, 53, 63, 92, 105,
    110

W

Waveform correlation. *See* Oxygen
    saturation; Pulse
Weight. determination/estimation, 9,
    24, 26
Wheezing, 19, 28, 32
  definition, 40
Work of breathing. *See* Breathing

X

Xiphoid process, 71
  avoidance, 72
  definition, 77

Additional Credits

Chapter 1
Figures 1-1, 1-3, 1-5, 1-6, 1-7, 1-8, and 1-10 © 2003 Nucleus Medical Art. All rights reserved. www.nucleusinc.com

Chapter 2
Figure 2-3 © 2003 Nucleus Medical Art. All rights reserved. www.nucleusinc.com

Figures 2-4, 2-5, 2-7, 2-8, 2-10, and 2-11 Courtesy of the National EMSC Slideset

Chapter 4
Figure 4-1 Courtesy of the National EMSC Slideset

Figures 4-2 and 4-3 © 2003 Nucleus Medical Art. All rights reserved. www.nucleusinc.com

Chapter 6
Skill Drill 6-1, Step 5 © 2003 Nucleus Medical Art. All rights reserved. www.nucleusinc.com

Figures 6-3 and 6-11 © 2003 Nucleus Medical Art. All rights reserved. www.nucleusinc.com

Chapter 7
Skill Drill 7-1, Step 7 © 2003 Nucleus Medical Art. All rights reserved. www.nucleusinc.com

Figures 7-2 and 7-19 Courtesy of the National EMSC Slideset

Figure 7-6 © 2003 Nucleus Medical Art. All rights reserved. www.nucleusinc.com

Chapter 8
Figure 8-5 Courtesy of Tomas B. Garcia, MD, FACEP

Figures 8-3, 8-6, and 8-9 © 2003 Nucleus Medical Art. All rights reserved. www.nucleusinc.com

Chapter 9
Figure 9-6 © 2003 Nucleus Medical Art. All rights reserved. www.nucleusinc.com

Unless otherwise indicated, illustrations for this book were created by Jones and Bartlett and Graphic World. Additional art was supplied by the authors, the Maryland Institute of Emergency Medical Services System, the American Academy of Orthopaedic Surgeons, and Jones and Bartlett Publishers.